CONQUERER
"My Journey with Cancer"

CONQUERER
"My Journey with Cancer"

by
Kathryn Brown

Copyright © 2014 by Kathryn Brown
All rights reserved. No part of this book may be reproduced, scanned, or distributed in any printed or electronic form without permission.
First Edition: November 2014
Printed in the United States of America
ISBN: 13-9781633184787

To My Sons James and Tevin, and my granddaughter Amiah,
You Mean The World To Me!

Acknowledgement

I am forever indebted to the following people for their help and support:

To my sister Val thank you for being there and helping through my battle.

To each and every one of my sisters and brothers of my church Gospel Tabernacle Outreach Ministries, I thank you for all of your help and support.

To my sisters thank you for being there and lending an ear to listen when I needed to talk.

To all my friends and co-workers thank you for all of your help and support during my most trying time.

THE TEST

Going through trials living this life, giving it my best at the end of it all asking God, "Did I pass the test?"
Insecurities may come, broken dreams no less, God has a lesson in the midst of it all
I sure hope I pass the test.
This God forsaken illness, taking my strength, my health, and sometimes my joy in life
But I know God will take my hand,
He will guide me through the strife.
Hold me close Lord through this mess
Help me focus on You, that I may pass the test.
Open my eyes so I may learn the lesson being taught, that my life may be pleasing in your sight
Restore tenfold what has been taken that I may
Enjoy the fruits of Your blessings with gratefulness and joy
Till I enter Your Glory on my day of rest
As I stand before You Lord, I pray You will say "My child you have passed the test."

Written by
Kathryn Brown

Journal 1

Wednesday, August 17, 2011
This is the day it all began. Waking up and getting Tevin off to intern camp. This was also my day to picket Verizon. Yeah, time to hit the pavement and show those greedy corporate hounds a thing or two, wanting to take away our benefits and stuff. Work stoppage here I come, but only for two weeks. After that a sistah has to look for other means of compensation. After dropping Tevin off at camp, I head to Taunton to fulfill my picketing assignment. I meet up with a few co-workers, walk in a circle in front of cars trying to get into the parking lot and saying a chant such as "What do we want? Contracts, when do we want it? NOW!!" This goes on for four hours, minus the bathroom run to McDonalds that takes about 45 minutes to an hour. Who can just walk into McDonalds and only use the bathroom? After my assignment, I drive home wondering when this strike will end. The August sun was too much I really missed going to work. Looking at the cars of people taking over our job. Parked in the lot, brought a bit of sadness to me, my car should be in that lot not theirs. This was the time I prayed extra hard for God to move on our behalf. I arrive at

home to an empty house and just sit in the living room listening to the silence and wondering how all this was going to pan out and who would eventually win in the end. Oh yeah, let me look at this mail on the couch, I thought. So I go over and began to open the first envelope. Wow! A bill under $100 can't beat that. Next envelope is opened and, "ouch" what was that sharp pain in my breast. I think nothing of it and continue opening the envelope, "ouch." There it is again and it is not stopping. The feeling of sharp needles begins to hit me continuously. When I realized it wasn't going to stop, I press my hand against my right breast to try and alleviate the pain and there it was, "BIG" as ever! Where in the world did that knot come from? How is it that I have never felt it before? I press against my breast again to confirm that what I felt is true. Yes, I have a knot the size of a golf ball in my right breast and I never knew it. Sounds crazy huh? I know, I know, how can something that big go undetected? I couldn't tell you the answer to that but I can tell you that because of how busy I was with work and school, it was very easy for me to neglect myself. Not to mention I have never given myself a self-breast exam nor have I ever went for a mammogram. Okay, now panic is setting in because I am on strike, I don't have an income coming in, I find a massive lump in my breast and at the end of the month I will not have medical coverage. Lord, I need you more like the wind in a hurricane. I jump on the phone to my sister who recommends me to an OB/GYN hospital. I call to make an appointment and the receptionist informs me they can schedule me for September. I quickly informed her why I am calling and that I will not have medical after the end of August. She quickly checks her schedule and puts me in for Monday, August 22, 2011. "Whew", Okay now I can get the ball rolling on this new discovery. What am I doing with a lump in my breast? This type of stuff doesn't happen to me. I'm used to seeing people on talk shows with this type of stuff, not me. Well, we shall see what happens next week. God, this is in your hands. You have never let me down so just take over, I have enough on my plate and I'm giving that to you as well.

This was the beginning of some of the most interesting and profound moments in my life. I welcome you on this remarkable journey and all the lessons, laughs, love and tears it brings. This journal is not only therapeutic for me but in some way I pray someone will find comfort in knowing that their petitions on my behalf were not in vain, that God was moving as their life was moving in prayer. I have embraced the well wishes, I have embraced the circumstances, and I have welcomed and embraced my duty to stand through it all and trust and believe that God is in control. Through adversity, through pain, through the storm, through MRI's, through CT scans, through biopsy's, bone scans and chemotherapy, the voice of Maya Angelo resonates with me when she states; "Still I rise." The voice of Dr. Martin Luther King will resonate with me when I can say to Cancer, "Free at last, free at last, thank God almighty I am free at last." But above all else, the Scripture in Isaiah 53:5 which states, "But he was wounded for our transgressions, he was bruised for our iniquities; the chastisement of our peace was upon Him and with his strikes I am healed."

Welcome to My Journey…….

Peace Be Unto You

Monday, August 22, 2011
Today I am on my way to the Doctor's office. I took a half day at work because of my doctor's appointment. My co-workers let me know not to worry. The lump is probably nothing and that

my doctor visit will be just a routine. They shared their stories of finding their own unwanted lumps and how everything turned out okay. Besides, they said, "You don't have any history of breast cancer in your family do you?" "No", I replied. Well that made me feel better knowing that since there is not history of breast cancer, I should be okay. Hey, I'm thinking way too much into this that I just passed the place. I turned around and find a parking spot in the parking lot of another medical center. I hope my car does not get towed and walk to the building where I will have my exam. Pretty easy to find, close to home, I like that. Okay, I just checked in, filled out some paper work and began reading a magazine. The office is pretty relaxed, very comfortable and the atmosphere was rather laid back. "Kathryn?" That's me! I jump up and follow the doctor's assistant to the examining room. We go through the usual routine of taking blood pressure and asking the normal questions about any illnesses and family history of illnesses. Then it's time for the dreaded "scale". Man! I wish I would have utilized my Gold's Gym more often. Gee Whiz!! Okay now I'm sitting on the examining table with that all to couture medical gown on, swinging my feet waiting for the doctor to arrive.

I found a magazine with a very interesting article and found myself hoping the doctor wouldn't come in until I had finished reading. To my surprise she didn't. In walks Dr. M. She's a cute doctor, new to the practice and very polite. She goes over my records with me and I notify her of my concern regarding my breast. After she examines me she refers me to their other department to take a mammogram and to have an ultrasound done. I leave feeling better that I had taken care of my concern. I hate sitting in the doctor's office. I am always on the go so to sit idle feels like a waste of time. Maybe that's why I pay so much for car repairs. Sitting at the mechanics is a dreading task for me as well. Okay I have the rest of the day to myself. Oh how sweet it is!

Friday, September 2, 2011
Today is my appointment for my first mammogram. They say you should have your first one at 40 years old but I never did. I'm 44 years old and feel pretty healthy. I hadn't felt any lumps beforehand so I thought I was okay. I arrive to the same building as my previous exams only on a different floor. We go through the usual routine and I am given another high fashion gown to change into. I begin to watch Regis & Kelly on television and began

to think what great jobs they had. "Kathryn," I hear from the doorway. The mammogram technician greets me and leads me to a rather cold room with a monstrous machine positioned in the corner. She informs me of how the testing will go and how I may feel uncomfortable but that is only because they want to get a complete and accurate test. She begins to position my right breast on a cold flat surface and for some strange reason I felt I was being put on the chopping block. She begins to pull a lever down over my breast and squeeze it really tight. She takes the picture of the image and positions me in another angle for yet another image. She lets me know that they have to squeeze a little more firmly because of the thickness of my breast and I began to wonder if she is off-handedly saying, "Your fat and so is your breast so we have to press harder." After the mammogram I am led into the waiting area again to have the ultra-sound done. About 10-15 minutes later, the same technician comes back and informs me she needs to take four more images of my right breast. Normally, I would have been a little irritated but the look on her face let me now this was something to be concerned about. After entering the room she informed me that the doctor ordered these extra images after studying my first set. I began to watch the technician as she was moving about the room and realized her whole body language was totally different. Her face showed concern and she moved about the room with a sense of urgency. I remain calm however, and made it through the second set of images wondering what will be the result when the doctor came in. I finally took the ultrasound and was informed by the technician to stay in the room and the doctor would be in to speak with me. I wait for about 15 minutes or was it 20? I'm not sure but thoughts of what that technician who administered the mammogram kept playing over and over in my head. "It's probably nothing," I told myself. Maybe she was reprimanded for not taking good pictures the first time. Yeah that's it!! That upset look on her face was from her being scolded by the doctor. All this is playing over and over in my mind until the doctor walks in. She is an older woman in her 50's but very professional in appearance. She has that look of experience and surety about her. Kind of like if she told you something, she knew what she was talking about because she was talking from experience. She asked me how I was doing and I told her I was doing well. She informed me that my image from the mammogram and the ultra-sound looked abnormal and that she was referring me for a biopsy and two other tests. One of which I remember being called a stereotactic. Can't remember the name of the other one though. I asked her about my images, something like, "what is the concern," and she straight forwardly told me that when I go for my biopsy, she expects my results to come back positive for cancer. Inwardly I was rattled but outwardly remained calm. She let me know my images were disturbing however, it was curable and not to worry. The office assistants led me to the office where I was given an appointment at women and infants hospital. Now the whole office has that look of concern and is moving with a sense of urgency. I began to realize the mammogram tech had taken good images after all. I leave the office with a bunch of good lucks and concerned looks from everyone and an appointment for a biopsy. I arrive at my car in the parking lot, thankful it hadn't been towed and just sit there wondering what had just happened. As I begin to drive, I can hear the doctor's voice say, "I am expecting your results to be cancerous." I begin to cry and get a little nervous; however, I do not let it settle in. I say a prayer and just let the day marinate in my mind. Me with cancer, No way!! I will be back in her office with her saying,

"Okay, I was wrong but we needed to take precautions anyway just to be on the safe side." Yeah, that's what's gonna happen. I don't have time for cancer. I could not have neglected myself that much where I could have let this happen. This is so not happening right now….

Monday, September 5, 2011
Today I told my supervisor about my experience at the doctors on Friday. As I was driving to work I thanked God again for the company and the union calling off the strike and allowing us to return to work while they worked through the contract. So we are still working under the old contract which allows me to have free medical. My supervisor seems a bit startled but reassures me everything will be okay. She lets me know about FMLA (Family Medical Leave of Absence) and prints out papers for me to have my doctor sign. I thank God for my supervisor Karen. She is so professional and every time we learn about leadership in class I think of her. I told my sister Val as well and she was pretty shocked as I was. I didn't want to tell any of my other sisters until I had a definite diagnosis. I told my cousin Anissa and she was very encouraging as well and let me know she was there for me no matter what. I still cannot believe I

11

am in this position right now. I am not anxious or worried and as a matter of fact I am rather calm about the whole thing. However, it just doesn't seem real. God, it's in your hands, cause I sure don't know what to make of all this.

<u>Tuesday, September 13, 2011</u>
Today is the day of my biopsy. I am not sure what to expect but I am ready for it. My sister Val comes to pick me up and we first take my son Tevin to school then we are off to Women and Infants Hospital. When we pull up to the hospital I find that they have valet parking. Oh snap!! That's a first for me. I've never seen anything like that before. Well we register at the front desk and make our way to the elevators. The floor we are headed for is zero. A zero floor? Isn't that usually called the basement? Anyway, once there I register again with the receptionist and we sit in the waiting area. Everything is beginning to feel real to me now. It's settling in that is something I am going through and will be a part of my life as another experience I can share with others. I look around the waiting area and I see women young and old sitting and waiting. Some with their loved ones others by themselves. I realized that some of the men in the waiting area

that escorted their wives or significant others to their appointments had looks of concern on their faces. Oh yeah, this was no ordinary waiting area, this was a whole new world. A world you could not leave with a doctor's prescription and his orders of bed rest. A world you could not leave in just a few days by taking it easy. A world you could not leave by taking cough medicine from your local drug store. This world bought fear to the average person and to the strong. This world bought urgent care to the patient and bought doctors together by the numbers. This world even startles mammogram technicians. Wow!! What have I allowed myself to get into? By neglecting my health, I have allowed myself unknowingly become a citizen of this world. So here I sit, waiting for my turn to take tests to see if I really belong here. "Kathryn," okay there goes my name again. My sister stays in the waiting area and I follow the assistant to a room where I change into yet again a high fashion gown and lock my belongings in a locker. I sit in another waiting area for about 5 minutes then I am led into a room where two other assistants greet me. They're very friendly and make me feel as if, I had known them before. One of the assistants was Lourdes. An older woman of Spanish decent, she speaks English well enough to be working at the hospital and her work ethic is fantastic. I automatically realized she had to show the staff she was worthy of being there regardless of her broken Spanish. I am lectured on the procedure which is called a stereotactic and I am shown now I will be laying on the bed once the procedure begins. The doctor comes in and he again goes over everything and asks me if I have ever seen my film that was taken which showed their concern in the first place. I tell him no and he tells me to come over to the screen on the wall where he proceeds to show me the area of concern. He says that because the mass is so large there is cause for alarm. He shows me a few calcium deposits then points to an area that looks like lightning bolts. He explains that this is the area of concern and is their main focus of urgency at hand. Okay so I crawl on the table and position myself on my stomach with my breast through a hole that is already in the bed. I am given local anesthesia and a few samples are taken from the tissue in my breast. Everything lasted about 20 or so minutes. I am taken into the waiting area again and I am wondering what the biopsy will be like. Well I didn't have to wait too long because I am escorted into a smaller room with a machine used for ultrasounds. I lay on the table face up and I am given more anesthesia. Several more samples are taken, this time with a device that has an annoying clicking sound. I began to think, "Of all the money given to medical research, they couldn't create a device that made less noise." Good grief! Now everything is over and I am wheeled back into the room I had just left so I could be bandaged up. The nurse tells me not to do any strenuous work and to just take it easy until tomorrow morning when I can remove my bandages before my shower. I am given extra bandages and ice packs to take home with me and a page of instructions to follow. I meet my sister out in the initial waiting area and she takes me to get something to eat in the cafeteria. Love that Cafeteria! Love my sister. She has a great heart and is always willing to help when she can. I'm glad she was there. I needed the company. We leave the hospital and she drops me off at home. It's quiet again but the silence is loud. I still feel a part of this other world but I am just not around the other citizens now. I am alone, set a part; I have been separated for a purpose. This world I'm in does not have to be as dark and gloomy as people make it out to be. I don't have to accept the gloom and doom of it all. I can still have the joy from the world I am use to, I can still have the peace that people do not understand and I can still have a smile that says everything is and will be alright. And mean it. Let me go to the one person who has given me all those things and has never taken them away. The one person who has entered this world with me and has never left my side since the beginning. Thank you God for being an ever present help in need.

Friday, September 16, 2011
Okay it's been three days since my biopsy and I am beginning to feel anxious. I know the Bible says to "be anxious for nothing," but Lord I can't help it. The staff and the hospital told me my results would take about a week to come back so they should have them to my doctor by the following Wednesday for my follow up appointment. All week my supervisor and my co-workers, (I have only told a few) are telling me not to worry. That everything will come back negative, they will remove the lump and I will be back to normal. I'm taking all of this in and using it to calm my anxiety. Then I began to wonder, God has always taken care of me. If this is something serious, He knows all about it and is working it out. He worked behind the

scenes to send us back to work when we were on strike thus giving me back my medical to take care of all this.
Yeah, I'm going to be alright. God saw I had a need and straightened everything out to my benefit. Okay I feel a lot better about things and return to my normal routine of the day. Sitting in front of my work computer e-mailing and working and wondering what's for lunch. I wonder what the lab has done with my results and how they have reacted if the results were positive and I shake my head trying to remove those thoughts and focus on the positive things. I feel as if I don't really need this to think about because there are so many other things I have to focus on but the enormity of it all will not leave my thoughts. Is it o.k. to think about this? Hey I may be Christian but I am also human. Of course it its o.k. just don't dwell. I order lunch and think about the weekend…

Wednesday, September 21, 2011
Okay I wake up today a bit anxious about my doctor's appointment. Today I get my results on my biopsy. I am a little concerned and anxious but I try to make myself feel that I am ready for any type of news be it good or bad. I take a half day at work and find myself speeding on the highway. Guess my foot

feels the anxiety as well. Finally I arrive at my doctor's office. I sit in the reception area for about 15 minutes until I hear my name called. I can hear the pounding of my heart in my ears as I walk to the examining room. I sit for what seems like forever and in walks Dr. M. She asks me how I feel and I let her know I feel just a little anxious about the results. She lets me know that the lab had not sent the results back but she would try to get them for me tomorrow. I sit there trying to stay poised but in my mind I am thinking "WTF!! What do you mean no results? It's been a week and a day." She apologizes but lets me know she will do the best she can. She gives me a number to call Women and Infants Breast Health Center. She lets me know to make the appointment ASAP. She apologizes once again and I leave her office feeling defeated for some reason. I wanted to know that I had beaten their predictions. I wanted to know that I had overcome the odds but instead I am driving home with nothing. I am ticked!!

Thursday, September 22, 2011
Today I am looking forward to calling my doctor. She had to have heard something since I left her office yesterday. I get to work and arrive to my anxious co-workers wondering what my

results were. I told them they hadn't come in and they show signs of shock and concern. I'm really not in the mood to talk about it so I just sit quietly at my desk until 10am. I call my doctor to see if my results had been received and I am informed that she was out of the office and would not return until the following Wednesday. After hanging up the phone, I have an inner dialect with myself, asks God to forgive my language and head back to my desk. To say I was upset would be an understatement. I begin to try and psych myself up again, trying to believe the tests will be negative and that God is giving me time to have more faith so He can prepare me for an awesome testimony. I don't know if that sounds logical but those were my thoughts and I'm sticking to them. Okay I just have to deal with the coming days until next week. I go back to work and think about two things that are pleasing and wonderful. Lunch and quitting time.

Friday, September 23, 2011
Today I made my appointment at the Health Center. I have an appointment with Dr. T. Okay don't ask me to say his name 3 times because I only know how to spell it by looking at the appointment card. Five more days until I get my results. Gee whiz!! I hate

this waiting game. Lord please help me!

Wednesday, September 28, 2011
Rise and shine girl!! Today is the day. I finally will get my results. I wonder which team will draft me? The positive team or the negative team. It doesn't matter, it's all good. God is on my side. I get to work before 9am and I want to call my doctor but I wait until 9:15 am. I get the receptionist who informs me the doctor is with a patient and that she will have her call me when she is finished. She informs me that my results are in but she was not able to give them to me because it was the doctor's position to do that. I told her I understand which I truly did and hung up the phone. Now the anxiety was in overdrive because I knew my results were in and things would change for the better or worse. I went back to my desk not really able to concentrate and looking continuously at my cell phone. Finally I couldn't take it anymore. I call again at 11:15 a.m. and I let the receptionist know that the wait for my results is driving me crazy. She lets me know that my doctor had been given my message and that she would be calling me but not to worry because if it was anything serious I would have gotten a phone call a while ago. After hanging up I began to

wonder if the receptionist should have told me that. If my results were positive she just fed me false hope. Then I began to wonder if she knew about my results and was inadvertently telling me everything was okay, God please!!! I just want to know. I go back to my desk yet again feeling as if I am chasing after something that no one wants to give me. Finally, after about 20 minutes my cell phone rings and the doctor's number shows up. I run to the hallway for better reception on my cell phone to answer the call and my doctor apologizes for not getting back to me sooner. She asks me if I had made the appointment at the Health Center and I quickly informed her I had and that my appointment was on October 11th. She tells me to make sure I keep my appointment because the news she had for me was not good. I began to hear my heart pound and I feel as if everything around me has gone silent. "Kathryn," she says, "the samples taken from the six o'clock position of your right breast came back negative for cancer, however, the samples taken from the 9 o'clock position came back positive for cancer." She apologizes for not having better news for me and lets me know that from here on I was in the hands of the Breast Health Center. She wishes me good luck, I thank her and the conversation ends. I go into a nearby conference room and just sit. Then the tears come, and they come, and they come some more. Tears filled with uncertainty, flowing. Tears filled with fear, flowing. I thought I was able to handle the news and face it head on. What I wasn't anticipating was the tone of voice in which the news was given. I know, I know I have to trust God in all things and I do. But right now I want the right to cry, I want the right to be concerned, I want the right to be scared, I want the right to say I am human first. Being a Christian doesn't mean we're super-human, being a Christian means we are aware we need someone higher and more powerful than us to get through this life. Right now I need all the higher power I can get. I wipe my eyes, go to the bathroom, clean my face and text my supervisor with the news. I take her up on her previous offer to go home early if the news wasn't great. I drive home in a daze not even knowing what to do next. Where do I go from here? I call my sister Val to tell her the news but as soon as she hears my voice she begins to tell me about how she removed a huge rock from her yard by blowing it up. After her talking for about 20 minutes or so she asks me what I called her for and I lie and say I forgot. At that point I just didn't feel like talking. I wait a while and text my cousin Anissa who calls me and encourages me. I just can't believe this day. Oh I forgot I have class tonight. I need the change of scenery and a different atmosphere right now. At break from class and I call my sisters in Atlanta to let them know. They are all shocked because of breast cancer not being in our family history. My sister Deneen begins to cry but I can't follow suit. I'm tired of crying at this point. I'm sure there will be plenty of time and opportunity for that. Okay I've told my sisters now for the main event. Telling my kids…

Monday, October 3, 2011
It's been five days since my diagnosis and I have been trying to process it all. I told my oldest son James who was shocked but I quickly informed him I would be okay. We sat on the bed in his room looking at the television and he affectionately laid his head on my shoulder. I let him know not to tell Tevin just yet and that I will do that in due time. I also let my friends and sisters in the Lord Jackie and Pat know. I ask them not to say anything because right now I don't understand nor have answers myself for all that is going on. They agree and I thank God for their friendship and loyalty. I also let my pastor know and she begins encouraging me as always. I don't

really go to my pastor for much because I know she has a lot on her plate and some of the stuff I hear people say they go to her about is truly unnecessary. Half the time I'm saying to myself, "Really? You needed pastor for that? Gimme a break!" Needless to say, when I do go to my pastor, it's for something I really, really need her guidance on. I decide to call another close person in my life. Sister Diane Dean. She has babysat Tevin since he was three months old and she and I have bonded ever since she also had breast cancer so she was the ideal person to talk to. She encourages me as well and lets me know that everything will be alright. After our conversation she prays with me and tells me she loves me. I can't wait for my appointment to find out more of what's going on and what they intend to do on my behalf. I guess it's just a waiting game from here…

Tuesday, October 11, 2011
Today I had an appointment with Dr. T. She examined me and said she was ordering another biopsy because she felt a lump under my arm. Lymph nodes they call it. After the exam she begins to talk with me about surgery and how it is inevitable, that it will happen. She lets me know that if I didn't need surgery I wouldn't be in

her office because she was a surgeon. She continues to let me know that the "tumor" was very large and that she was going to refer me to a colleague of hers named Dr. S. We continue to talk a bit and she tells me of a group at the hospital that meets once a week and it consists of other women with the same issues as me. I am introduced to a counselor named Carrie who further explains the program to me. After speaking with her I ask my doctor how long did she think the "tumor" had been there and she informed me it was there for a very long time. She asked me if I had ever had a mammogram and I informed her I had not and she said if I had went for one they could have detected it a long time ago. She said because the growth was on the meaty side of my breast it would have been hard for me to detect it when it was smaller but a mammogram would have picked it up. She reassured me that they are helping me now so not to worry. However she has no idea how much she has validated how I have felt all along. That I have been neglectful in caring for myself. I have neglected the body God has given to me. I have neglected the medical attention it should have had and the nutrition attention it needs. God I am so sorry. Help me to do better in caring for the things you have entrusted me with. I leave the examining room with the counselor and she gives me her card, leads me to a desk to make an appointment with Dr. S and lets me know to call her with any questions. I thank her, we shake hands and I am given an appointment with Dr. S for the next day. I leave the office feeling as if I am in good hands but a little overwhelmed at the same time. As I pull out of the parking lot I feel as if this building is going to be my second home for a very long time...

Wednesday, October 12, 2011
Today I had an appointment with Dr. S. He is a very noble man I can tell, yet very knowledgeable and I later learned he is one of the top doctors in his field. He goes over my chart with me and then he himself examines me. After the examination he informs me that upon research of my breast cancer, it has been determined that I have a grade 3 type of cancer which is very aggressive. He lets me know that it has been determined that I will need chemotherapy and then surgery. He further states that ordinarily they would be able to treat breast cancer with a milder form of treatment, but that would only have been if it was detected at an early stage. However in my case, because the cancer passed the early stage and is so aggressive they

have ruled out the milder forms of treatment and will need to do chemotherapy. Additionally, I will need chemo once a week for four months. This will give them time to try and shrink the tumor before surgery. I was further informed they would have done surgery first then chemo, but due to the size of the tumor, surgery would be very extensive. This is why they wanted to shrink the tumor first then do the surgery. I was also told I would be given something called Herceptin. This would work along with the chemo in helping to shrink the tumor. He said in some cases the tumor shrank considerably and sometimes surgery was not even needed but that all cases were different. He asked me if I had any questions and I asked him about the drugs and chemo having any side effects and he said that Herceptin had little to no side effects, however chemo will probably make me nauseous, I will probably lose my hair and I might get a tingling feeling in my fingers and toes. If that should happen I was to let him know because that is a sign of me being susceptible to infection. He also said he would be able to give me something for nausea if I should ever need it. We end our session and I am led yet again to the appointment desk. I have appointments for four more tests all to be taken in one day. I leave the building yet again with my head reclining with all that is going on, trying to process it all. "I need an appointment book," I say to myself. I have a feeling this is just the tip of the iceberg...

Friday, October 14, 2011
I am excited about the dance jam at my church tonight. Every year it gets better and better. I love how God uses my fellow brothers and sisters in Christ to minister in dance. After work I rush home to pick up Tevin, stop at Burger King and off to church we go. We arrive early, of which I am glad, so I find a seat that is pretty much near the front. I am reminded that after the Dance Jam, there is all night prayer. I can't stay because I have Tevin with me and frankly I forgot. As the program begins I am in awe of the amount of detail that went into preparing for this night. There are guest dancers from Christ Temple Church that are just as anointed. Sis Margie dances but not before dedicating her dance to me. What a beautiful dance it was. I run downstairs in the bathroom crying like a baby. At the end I thank her for her thoughtfulness and she lets me know I am always in her prayers. I return home and try to watch television while laying on my couch. I should have known better. That is a lethal

combination. I finally get into a good sleep when all of a sudden the phone rings. I jump automatically thinking of my son James who was out with friends that night. When I look at the caller I.D. I realized it was Sis. Pat. "Why in the world is she calling me at 12:30 a.m." I'm thinking. I answer the phone and she begins to tell me how pastor had let everyone out early because God had given everyone the answer they were looking for. She then proceeds to tell me that she believes God is going to dry up the cancer in my breast and that I need to jump up and down right now and thank Him. She is telling me like she was a radical evangelist on television that I usually turn from without a second thought. She begins to scream and shout hallelujah and again tells me I need to get out of bed and jump up and down and thank God for my healing right now. I ask her where she is and she proceeds to tell me she is on her way to IHop with a few people. She said that pastor wanted them to yell out a person's name that they wanted Him to heal and she told me she yelled out my name. OKAY now I'm pissed because I asked that heifer not to say anything. Now she has peaked everyone's curiosity. Whenever she has told me something I have always been true to her wishes not to say anything, so for her to go and call my name out was a slap in the face. I know her intentions were good but they should have been better and she should have kept her mouth shut. Our conversation ends and I hang up the phone pretty annoyed. One because she woke me up with all that deranged yelling and two because she hadn't honored my wishes. Now I have to set the record straight with her but do it in a loving way. I don't want her to think it is alright for her to continue doing what she did so I have to nip it in the bud quickly. I am not ready to face the inquiring mind of people that are wondering what is wrong with Sis. Kathy? You had better believe I will keep my mouth shut from now on!!

Saturday, October 15, 2011
Today I have an echo-cardiogram at local Hospital. My sister Val and I get there around 9:25 a.m., five minutes before my appointment and we sit in the waiting area. I begin to read an article in the magazine but I am called into the examining room for the procedure. It was quite simple and painless and the technician and I struck up a great conversation the whole time. This test was to determine the condition of my heart before beginning chemo. I leave the hospital with the whole day ahead of me. I'm

not use to having a whole weekend to myself. What will I ever do??

Sunday, October 16, 2011
Today I arrive at church pretty early and I am able to get a few things done in the office. I remember Sis. Maggie needs tithing envelopes so I quickly make her a few out and head out to the sanctuary. I see her standing at her seat in the front row so I head over to her and hand her the envelopes. She thanked me for them and then embraces me and begins to thank God over and over in my ear. "What in the world is going on?" I wonder. She has never done this before. Then it hits me. She was with Pat that early Saturday morning when Pat called me with all that yelling. I thought I heard a voice in the background and I thought it sound like Sis. Mag but I didn't say anything. Now it was confirmed. Okay I'm not only ready to slap the taste out of Pat's mouth, but anything else she feels she needs to say but shouldn't. I walk to my seat feeling as if I do not need to be singing in the praise team because I am pretty bound up right now. I say a prayer and get through service by the will of God. Once I get home I make it my business to call Pat to let her know I do not appreciate her calling my name out at all night prayer. I do not mention the

fact about my gut feeling of her telling Sis. Mag because that's one less thing I need for her to tell. Pat agrees and says she understands and I leave it at that. I hang up the phone realizing why I do not have too many people around me and why I keep my business to myself. I know Pat meant well, and I certainly do not want to take away the fact that she has been there for me and my kids. Not to mention, she has a heart of Gold, but right now I need to process a lot of things and knowing I have someone's trust would be comforting right now…

Tuesday, October 18, 2011(Morning Entry)
Today I am preparing to have four, yes; four tests done today at the Medical Hospital.
I had to drink two bottles of some milky substance with a hint of berry flavor for my CT scan. I arrive at the doctor's office and I am whisked right in amidst other people that I 'm sure have been there way before me. I change into a gown, and go into a room with a huge machine that will perform the scan. After that I am whisked to another room where I will be given my first ever MRI. I have to lie face down which is okay with me because I am unable to see that I am inside a machine thus eliminating

claustrophobia. After that I wait a while and then I am whisked off for an ultrasound. All these procedures do not take too long however I remember my last test which was another biopsy that Dr. T ordered when she examined me the last time. I am instructed to return at 1 p.m. so I go and have lunch at their awesome cafeteria! At 1 p.m. I return for my biopsy and I am led into a room with a machine used for mammograms. The doctor arrives, introduces herself and lets me know what she will be doing. During the procedure, I am able to see her taking samples from the lymph nodes under my arm which I found to be really cool. Afterwards, the rest of the day was mine. Well not really I had school.

Tuesday, October 18, 2011 (Evening Entry)
I arrive home from school and found Tevin home with all the lights on. Doesn't this boy know I pay for electricity? Kids have no sense of frugality. I go into the kitchen and automatically God lets me know that now is the time to tell Tevin about my diagnosis. I try to rationalize that I just walked in the house and that I will do it later but there really is no arguing with God. When He tells you to do something just do it. Well I go into the living room and I let Tevin

know I have something to tell him. His eyes automatically get big and he says, "Is it about me?" I tell him "no" and began to wonder what he did in school that I should know about but he is not telling me. I make a mental note to check his book bag for any notes and the voicemail for any messages. We sit on the couch and I began to tell him that I have been going to the doctor a lot because I have been sick. I realize I now have his undivided attention when I mention I was sick so I let him know that I went to the doctor and they told me I had breast cancer. At first he didn't believe it but when I assured him it was true I could see the look of concern on his face and that he wanted to cry. I quickly let him know that I was going to be o.k. and that the doctors said it was curable so don't worry. After our talk he sat on the couch stunned and said, "I can't believe my own mother has breast cancer." He lets me know that because October is breast cancer awareness month they were talking about it a lot in school. He seemed pretty calm after our talk and he wanted to get some breast cancer bracelets over the weekend. I ask him about how he would feel if my hair fell out during my chemo treatments and he said I would just have to get some wigs. My kids are the best!!!

Conquerer "My Journey with Cancer"

Wednesday, October 19, 2011
Today I had a 2:30 p.m. appointment with doctor S. He informed me that the tumor in my breast was larger since my last visit. Before it was 3cm but since the other tests, they realized that it was 5cm. He called over to Women and Infants for the results of my tests I took yesterday and informed me that the lymph nodes under my arms were in fact cancerous as well. I am curious to know how cancer is formed and he explains that the body functions like a sewage system. He says the arteries flush out all the bad stuff while the veins process the good stuff, however when the arteries do not flush out the bad stuff, it causes a backup in the body and when it is not taken care of it causes cancer. I hope I am explaining it right. He was better at it than I am. He lets me know he would also like to try an experimental drug on me that would work in conjunction with the Herceptin and chemo. This drug worked on some people but not on others. It also will help with putting a stop the growth of the tumor. He explains in detail everything about the drug and what research has found with other participants. He gives me a hand-out with several sheets of paper and encourages me to read about it further. Afterward I am introduced to an RN named Heather who further lets me

know about the study and what it entails. I am given an appointment with her for Oct 25 to further go over everything regarding my chemo procedure. She encourages me to have questions available and to bring someone along for reinforcement, however she ensures me by the end of our session all my questions will be answered. Boy! She's good...

Thursday, October 20, 2011
Today I had a good day at work. It was pretty slow but nonetheless it was good. I went to speak with a co-worker of mine named Pat Baker. I like Pat. She is an older woman in her mid 50's but very nice and approachable. She is one of the co-workers I confided in about my diagnosis. Well on this particular day I walk over to her desk located on the other side of the building. Her area is called "Mahogany Row" by the other people in the building. She and I begin to talk and she asks me how I am feeling and I give her an update on all. I have been going through with all the appointment and everything. I tell her about the other lymph nodes they found to be cancerous and she begins to have a very sad look on her face. She asks me if I told my kids and I began to tell her about how I told Tevin and she begins to try her best to hold back tears.

She wasn't good at it and neither was I. We hug each other and she squeezes me tight to let me know I will be alright. I kiss her on the cheek and thank her and walk back to my desk with a feeling of knowing I have just been shown some genuine love from a co-worker. And I thought this was going to be just another ordinary day...

Friday, October 21, 2011
Today I had a bone scan done to make sure there were no cancerous cells within the bones. It took about 45 minutes for the whole test and I was told to wait in the room while the doctor examined the film. The technician comes in again and says the doctor would like pictures of the lower part of each leg. Deja Vu all over again. Hey at this point nothing surprises me. He takes a few more scans and I leave. My sister Val is waiting for me so I drive her to her car and go home. I was told things will slow down after all these tests. I sure hope so...

Tuesday, October 25, 2011
What a day it is. I began my appointment at Women and Infants Breast Health Center for my chemo talk. My sister accompanies me and we ask questions and receive very informative information the nurse, Heather has a

great sense of humor and is very forth coming with information. We make more appointments, blood work, another biopsy and another scan of my fibula, the lower part of my legs, all of which will produce better film for the doctor to examine. I have realized I am tired of all these tests now. I'm tired of going back and forth. I'm tired of waiting for results. I just want to get on with the treatments.

Wednesday, October 26, 2011
I had a brief appointment with Dr. S today and he went over my appointments with me. He is a very interesting doctor and I love his analogies of everything. I may be starting chemo later than expected but I just want to get the ball rolling. In due time I guess…

Monday, October 31, 2011
Today Is Halloween and here I sit in the doctor's office getting yet another biopsy. This afternoon I also begin my "Herceptin run in" which is before my chemo which is to begin Nov 18th. I just want all the appointments to stop and for the treatments to begin. There is so much going on I miss being normal. I still have my peace within but I also miss normal. I thank God for staying by my side and keeping me through all this. I guess this is the

new normal until my full recovery. I'll just settle in and let God lead the way!!!

Monday, October 31, 2011- 1 p.m.
Here I sit getting my Herceptin run-in. The atmosphere is pretty tranquil and the staff is really nice. My nurse Rosa is dressed as Princess Lea from the Star-Wars. Her costume is very impressive. I sit for 1 ½ hrs. My sister and I, and we watch Family Feud with Steve Harvey. I love this show now that he is on it. They give me lunch and a snack and I feel like the center of attention. I'm treated well here at the doctor's office. It makes this journey much easier to bear. Thank you God...

Tuesday, November 1, 2011
Today I had an appointment with my surgeon Dr. T. She explained to me about how she was going to surgically insert a port for my treatments which will all make it easier to administer the chemo and Herceptin without having to stick me with a needle every time. Afterwards I met with Heather the nurse who went over all my appointments with me. She's the best! I love her spirit. She went to get an email that Dr. S sent her regarding my appointment and she told me she had all the office gossip about me in her email. I

laughed but really wanted to say, "Really? So what does it say? Was I switched at birth? Am I really a man? Am I Dr. S's love child" But I kept my cool and saved the jokes for later. I feel I am really going to need a sense of humor in the coming weeks…

Friday, November 4, 2011
These days have been going by so quick and sometimes I feel lost and confused. So many appointments, so many things to remember and so little time for it all. Next week will be the first week. I will not have any appointments. Oh yeah, I forgot, I have one Friday but it is in the evening. I know I will look back on all this and see a reason for it all. I'll see why God chose me to go through this and see what it is I have learned and how I have spiritually grown. But right now, in the midst of it all, I am just trusting God to bring me out. I am looking to Him from whence cometh my one and only help because I will need it in the coming months…

Wednesday, November 9, 2011
Today is the second day I have been fighting a cold. I am trying to overcome these symptoms because I have surgery on Monday to have a "port" implanted so I can begin chemo next Friday. I am beginning to feel a bit

anxious now, only because I am uncertain as to how I will react to the chemo. Yeah I was given the "run down" about all the side effects but I'm not too sure if I am ready for my hair to fall out. I'm going to the hair dresser this week but my sister is telling me I am wasting my money. The nerve of her! I don't want to walk around waiting to go bald. Besides, I don't know how long it will take for that to happen if at all. I'll take my chances and get my hair done anyway. Also, school will be ending for the semester next week and I am so glad. This semester was very challenging for me because I have been trying to keep up with the work and trying to keep my doctor appointments as well. I think I've done well but I will be taking the winter semester off. It may set me back a bit as far as graduation is concerned but that's okay. My health is important. God bless!!!

<u>Monday, November 14, 2011</u>
Today I have my port inserted to prepare me for chem... I am anxious to get everything started and see the results. I have to be at the hospital at 7 a.m. However surgery takes place after 9 a.m. Not sure what to expect but I put my trust in God and God alone...

Monday, November 16, 2011
I am feeling a little better after the surgery. My body is really sore so I am trying to take it easy. Surgery went well however. I kept falling back to sleep because of the anesthesia. Then they send me home with Vicodin. Really? Oh well. I have to do something to alleviate the pain. I haven't taken the bandage off yet but will do so tomorrow the day before chemo. What a whirlwind this whole thing has been. I thank God for my sister Valerie. She has been a true Godsend through all this. She has been there for my appointments and has fixed dinner for my kids and me every night. God bless her. She has a good heart. I thank God for my kids as well they have been troopers through all this and have also been very helpful and supportive. I see God in everything that is said and done so I know he is walking beside me through all this. Thank you Jesus!!

Friday, November 18, 2011
Today I had my first round of chemo. It went well although I was concerned about the needle going through my skin into the port. I was there for about 6 ½ hours because of my blood work not being done. I had to do that then wait for about two hours for the results. I remember seeing a girl of about twenty-

something coming in there for chemo and realizing how diverse this disease really is. I met a woman during my chemo who told me she had been battling pancreatic cancer for three years. Wow!! What a blessing because that is a deadly form of cancer that a lot of people do not get to see three years of their life after being diagnosed. I left today realizing how truly good God is and that all things are in his hands. Praise God!!

Monday, December 5, 2011
Happy Thanksgiving! I am in a new apartment and am loving it. My sister Val and sis Diane Dean said they hated my house but love my apartment. Now they tell me. My boys and I will be going to Martha Dean and James house for dinner so I will not have to worry about cooking. I am thankful for my very life even though I have suffered a setback. I am thankful for my children, their health and for them being good kids. I thank God for my sister Val who has been a true Godsend through all of this. She has been so dependable, so trustworthy and so available and I truly thank and praise God for her and her servants' heart. I thank God for my family, (church and biological), friends and coworkers who truly care for me and about me. I especially thank God for my pastors who

are truly followers of Jesus Christ and have his heart as their heart. I have so much to be thankful for that I cannot tell it all, however, God knows my heart. Praise His Holy name!!

Friday, November 25, 2011
Today I receive my second dose of chemo. Not really sure how I feel today but would like to be somewhere else besides here. I feel as if I have so much to do and so little time to do it. But first things first okay time for my chemo to start. Lord, have your way…

Monday, November 28, 2011
Today is my first day back to work and although I am excited to have some normalcy in my life I am a little apprehensive. About what? I have no idea I feel as if I have been sheltered for the past two weeks and now I am branching out on my own. I woke up feeling nauseous so I took my medication which worked in about 1 hour. Driving seemed foreign although I knew where I was going. I felt as if I was returning to work as a different person. Since leaving the job two weeks ago, I had the "port" inserted and I had to recover from that then I began my first chemo treatment. Not to mention there was the holiday however in-between I began feeling the change

within my body since beginning chemo. Fatigue, constipation, nausea and more fatigue. I keep checking to see if my hair is beginning to fall out however I am going to try and stop checking. If it happens it happens. I know I will be rid of this someday so I am just going to keep a positive attitude through it all. I know I will be able to help someone someday who may be going through the same thing. I want to be a blessing to them so I have to stay strong, be vigilant and fight the enemy at every turn. Lord, thank you for the strength.

Monday, December 5, 2011
Today was good day for me although I felt a bit tired. Work went well however my supervisor is suggesting I go out on FMLA. I tend to get ill at work and have to leave early at times. She is suggesting I should save my energy for other things and not waste it at work. I just want to try and maintain my normal routine. My doctor informed me at my last exam that the tumor is shrinking so that is truly a blessing. Just want all this to be over but until then to God be the glory!!!

Sunday, December 18, 2011
Today is the Sabbath and for the first time I do not feel like going to

church. I have been feeling sick in my body and very nauseous for over a week. However, I am going and I know God has a message for me. Also, my two co-workers, Kris and Annette are coming. They expect to see me there so that is another inspiration as well. So much is happening with my body and there are days I just want to stay in bed but again I just want to maintain some type of normalcy in my life. I despite this sickness I have and the nausea that comes with it. Everything stinks when I smell it and that also is a "thorn in my side." God I apologize for putting such a taxing burden on my body. It is because of my own negligence this has happened and for that I apologize. On another note, there is only one week until Christmas and I am not in the spirit at all. I just want everything back to normal. I'm sick of chemo, I'm sick of blood work, I'm sick of being sick…I'm just sick of everything. Yes, frustration is beginning to settle in and it is hard not to entertain it especially when you have to get on with life. Maybe trying to maintain normalcy isn't the way to go. Maybe I should try to be in the moment and just accept my current position and live with it until it is all over. Have I checked out of reality and didn't know it? Have I checked out of my previous self and not know it? God help me please!! Help me to take one day at a time. Help me to stay strong. Please take away this uncomfortable feeling and give me back my joy and peace. I don't seem to have that anymore. I feel it slipping away and I need it to maintain my peace of mind. Help me God, please.

Wednesday, December 28, 2011
Well, I went to the doctor today and was informed that my white blood cells were very low so I will have to skip my chemo treatment for this week. I have been given a prescription for medication that I have to take for three days in a row. I had planned a family trip for April 2012 but wasn't sure if I would be able to make it but my doctor informed me I could go so I am happy about that. Overall, the check-up went well, except for my cell count but Lord, I know I will be alright for by your stripes I am healed!!!

Sunday, January 1, 2012
Whew! Another year has come and gone. Where did the time go? So much has happened this past year Lord but through it all you have sustained me. Lord I thank you for the latter part of the past year because you have truly ministered to me about not only myself but about people I have let into my

life. I guess I trust a little too much and I give of myself too much even though it is not being reciprocated. I have trusted someone with information that I didn't want known at the time, and yes they knew this, however they disregarded my wishes and did the opposite. Now Lord, I am not really as upset at my business being told as I am of being betrayed by someone I thought to be a friend. I have kept their private matters that were entrusted to me just that, private but I guess they did not feel the same way. But God, I am so glad for your Holy Spirit and your guidance and how to handle this whole situation. What's done is done. It cannot be taken back nor can it be changed but now I know how to handle things. Thanks to your Holy Spirit I know what can be shared and what cannot be shared. I still consider this person to be a friend but the level of friendship is not there anymore. Since my diagnosis, I have had things revealed to me that I shouldn't have seen before but more than likely chose to ignore because it was close to my heart and too painful to bear. Another person close to me has just distanced themselves and hasn't really been there like they use to. It seems as if since my diagnosis I have been the one reaching out to them and trying to maintain the friendship and getting nothing in return. I really valued this friendship for years and thought they did as well but now I know I have to move on and let bygones be bygones. I have to concentrate on myself and my health. Not to mention my relationship with Jesus. The other two pale in comparison to this relationship. I have noticed that the longer I have been saved the further life tries to pull me away from the Father. Family, work, school they are all deterrents that has been trying to pull me away from my "First Love." But I am so glad for your Holy Spirit Lord. I thank you for showing me the error of my ways. Thank you for showing me I do not have to do all things that come into my life and think I can still maintain a healthy and prosperous relationship with you. Not everything is a "God-thing" even in prosperity. Sometimes prosperity can cause one to be separated from the Father. Then again, that is not Godly prosperity but worldly-prosperity. Lord, I miss the time when I lived simply. I miss the times when my spirit was so open to you I woke-up excited about what was in store and what I was going to learn about you that day. I miss the times when your voice and spirit guided me without interruption. I miss my time with you. I miss that hunger and thirst I had when I first came to you.

Yes, I miss it but I will get it back. The enemies' camp will be missing some inventory because my joy will not be on the shelf, my love will not be in the frozen section and my peace, health and Godly prosperity will not be at the check-out counter. I am going back to the simple things in life where God can reach me more easily and where my access to Him is more open. Thank you God for that revelation over these past few days. Now I know where my concentration must life. Not on people because I know the arm of flesh will fail me but these relationships are not as important as my relationship with the Father. I look forward to this coming year and what is in store for me. I know my healing is one but I am excited to get back to the simple life and be with the Father without boarders in the way, once again. Yes, it will be a very Happy New Year!!

Monday, January 2, 2012
Today I have been thinking about my chemo treatment this Friday. I had to skip last week because of my low white blood cell count. My nurse Sandra was concerned about me going out for the New Year because I am susceptible to infection. I asked her what was my blood count and she informed me that a normal count is supposed to be '1500' but in my case I was only a '400'. She

let me know that if I felt a cold or any other symptom of an infection to treat it right away. She let me know which cough medicines to take and if for any reason I was unsure or I had any questions that I could call the center and speak with someone. I realize I have begun to count down the days until my final chemo treatment. I believe my doctor said the last one will be March 16th. Believe me it cannot come fast enough. I am going to need this vacation in April after all I have endured, mentally, physically and emotionally. Lord, I am going to need an extra dose of your strength because the last time I had chemo I was extremely nauseous and sick. The medication did very little to help so please spare me what I endured last time. Not to mention my sense of smell was totally off the charts. I hated every smell in my house including all cleaning agents. I had to walk around my house with a mask on because I hated the smells. However, I did find relief at the grocery store when I went food shopping. I wasn't bothered with any unpleasant odors so even after my cart was full and I was ready for check-out I just walked around the store because the air was so clean. I know things will get better…I'll just wait upon the Lord to renew my strength that I may soar like the eagles…yes, to soar like the eagles where the air is fresh and clean…I'll keep that vision, for without it, my Bible tells me I will perish and that I do not have room for…on another note I have been going back and forth about people who know about my diagnosis and people who don't that includes people in my family and people in my church. I really don't' know why I am writing about this but since I have decided to keep a journal once I was diagnosed I told myself part of my recovery would be to be honest with my feelings. There were people in my family that were told and there were people in my family that were not told. Not because I didn't want them to know but because they were not the ones I was thinking about telling at the time. The same was for my church family. There were people I told and then there were people I didn't tell. I only told certain people because I was close to them. They were told at the beginning stages of my diagnosis, during a time in which I didn't have all the answers and neither did the doctors. They were asked not to say anything only because I needed prayer and not inquisitive minds. I am not a person who really cares to have anyone know about what is going on in my life because I am and always have been a very private person. However, I'm sure there are going to be people who will be offended by me not telling them or wondering why I didn't say anything to the church so the church can pray for Sis. Kathy. Well I have come to find out that the whole church is not always on one mind and one accord. I have never been once to connect to the masses so if something needs to be done I know that only a few people are needed. Wow God! You are so good. As I am writing this journey, God has revealed to me that just like He chose the twelve and there was a betrayer amongst them, so was the case with the people I have chosen. The confidant became the betrayer (and shared information they should not have) but I thank God for his continued insight and wisdom through it all. I cannot lose my focus because that is what the enemy wants. I cannot have another type of cancer, hatred, eating away at me. This is just another part of me the journey, a learning process and I hope I have passed the test. I am so trying to keep everything around me simple and peaceful because things can go horribly wrong quickly and my continued focus on God and my recovery are at the forefront of my mind. Whew! Now that I have gotten that off my chest I feel better and can concentrate more freely and move forward…Forging ahead until the next entry…Praise God!

Sunday, January 8, 2012

Sitting at work today feeling very irritated and sleepy. Just wanting everything to be done and over with. I want normalcy again. It seems just when things are claiming down something else happens. It seems I get irritated easily now and I just want to be by myself. Well, I've wanted that before my diagnosis so now it's even more desirable. Not to mention I have found out that I am going through early menopause because of the chemo. It may continue after my treatment or it may stop. I will just have to wait and see. The hot flashes are getting on my nerve and sometimes I just want to rip my hormone out. Well, it's almost quitting time and I thought I was going to the gym after work but I lied to myself. Going home, taking off my gym clothes and sit in front of the television for the rest of the night. Lord please gets me home safely because fatigue is setting in really fast.

Monday, January 9, 2012

Today I slept all day. I woke up with the intentions on going to work but it didn't happen. I got dressed, took Tevin to school, and came back home and called my supervisor to tell her I will not be in. She tells me if I am not feeling well tomorrow to take it off as well. I hope into bed feeling very fatigued and weak. I slept for four hours straight. I can't remember the last time I laid in bed and slept the whole morning. I could have continued to sleep but I had to get up and get something to eat. I fixed eggs and biscuits and hopped right back into bed and slept some more. My nurse told me I would be fatigued after chemo but this is more than that. I feel as if I have no strength. I am trying not to give in to this feeling of being helpless. There are times I just want to be alone with no one around and nothing to do. I pray those aren't signs of depression. I am not claiming that one bit. I have too much to do and too far to go in my recovery to entertain that. I have to concentrate on the things that will keep me motivated, like my children and my family. I have a life to live. I can't give up now. This is not the end. God has shown me that this disease is curable, why am I walking around with a whoas-me attitude? Okay now I have to give myself the pep-talk. The type of encouragement I am standing on through this all. The scripture that makes it all worthwhile: Isaiah 53:5; Praise God. "But He was wounded for our transgressions, He was bruised for our iniquities; the chastisement of our peace was upon Him; and by His stripes we are healed."

Wednesday, January 18, 2012
Sitting here waiting for Dr. S to examine me and while I am doing so I am watching Dr. Oz. He is informing everyone about fungus that is found in orange juice imported from Brazil. Okay I went food shopping last week and bought a gallon of that stuff. I don't really know If it's imported or not but do I really need a fungus taking up residence in my body? Gee whiz! I am trying to get rid of what's been harboring in my body in my body for God knows how long and now I am being told I should be concerned about a fungus. Oh, by the way, although the FDA is aware of this, they are not recalling any orange juice that has already been imported into the United States. O.K. it's time to become agriculturally inclined and grow my own food. This is ridiculous!!

Friday, January 27, 2012
I am in the waiting area waiting to have chemo hoping I do not get as sick as I did the last time. I was very nausea and the smell of everything stunk. Last time I had to throw away all the air fresheners and although I had my furniture cleaned I hated the smell of that as well. The deal-breaker was when I went to KFC and bought a bucket of chicken. After putting the chicken in my car I began

to realize that the smell of marijuana was all too prevalent. I began to look around out the windows thinking someone around me was smoking it but there were only empty parked cars. I looked at the bucket of chicken and sniffed the bag it was in and lo' and behold there it was. My bucket of KFC smelled like a Bob Marley tour bus. I immediately began to roll the windows down thinking my illusion was going to give me a contact. When I got home I didn't want to bring the bucket in but as I sat in the car I had to remind myself that my sense of smell was only due to the effects of the chemo and that the chicken was safe to bring in the house and eat. What an experience that was! Well, needless to say, when I leave this session of chemo I will not be going to KFC. I think I will stay away from the chicken all together and make pork chops instead. Besides, I think I will be okay because my doses will be reduced today. I was told my platelets were low, which is expected so they will reduce my doses to try and bring them up to a normal level. This is the reason I began bruising while going for blood work. Large red bruises began to appear on my arm yesterday after giving blood work so my nurse told me my platelets were the reason for this. I thank God for His strength through all this for I know better days are ahead.

My eye is on the prize; I have tunnel vision; regardless of what my situation brings I know God will see me through; I am being refined in the fire and when it is all finished I will emerge pure as gold…Hey, I just met the best dog ever. His name is 'Angie' and he is a black Labrador retriever of 3 years. He is used as a therapy dog for the cancer patients here at the center. What a beautiful dog! He even has been taught to say his prayers which is what his trainer had him to do before leaving the room where I was having chemo. How awesome is that? God bless Angie's owner for sharing his beautiful animal with the patients of Women & Infants Breast Health Center. Angie, you're the best. Hope to see you again soon.

Friday, February 3, 2012
Today Sister Fran came with me to the chemo treatment. I was really glad she was there and we talked about some of everything during the five hours we were there. I really enjoyed her company and she was very encouraging as well. She prayed with me before my treatment and from there it was non-stop conversation. After my treatment, as I was driving home I was in high spirits but I also felt faint in my body and fatigue began to settle in. I began to wish I had taken Sis. Fran up

on her invitation to pick me up but instead I told her I would meet her there. I prayed all the way home that God would sustain my driving ability until I got home. As soon as I walked through the door I changed into my lounge wear a.k.a. sweat shirt and sweat pants and just laid on the couch. My body began to ache as well, I guess from the effects of my Neupogen shots to boost my white blood cells. Dec. Lenny was helping me with that because I just couldn't stick myself but praise God I have been able to do it myself now. Deacon Lenny and Sister Jenn are awesome. Their so supportive and understanding. To God by the glory. I have the best church family anyone can ask for…

Saturday, February 11, 2012
Today I can eat a decent meal without making myself do it. The nausea I feel after chemo is really unbearable. After my doctor's appointment yesterday he let me know that I can reduce my doses of Neupogen from three days to two. Praise God!! It's all about Him…chemo went well on Friday and I have to admit God really blessed me with an awesome staff at the Women and Infants Breast Health Center. My nurses' name is Sandra and she is just the best. She has the best smiling eyes and such a pleasant demeanor about

her. Her sense of humor is great as well. During my last visit while I was waiting for my treatments to start, she walks through the corridor with bags of carboplatin in her hands exclaiming, "chemo for everyone." I began to laugh because she sounds like the ice cream man walking in with a treat for everyone. Oh yeah, by the way, I have six more weeks to go before the end of my treatments. Praise God!! What began on November 18, 2011 will end on March 23, 2012. After getting that bit of news from my doctor I developed tunnel vision. I'm not looking to the left nor the right but forward to the finish line. To God Be All the Glory!!!

Saturday, March 3, 2012
Today was a very good day. I went out with a few of the single ladies in my church and we did a dinner and a movie. We saw Tyler Perry's movie "Good Deeds," then we went to T.G.I. Fridays. The fellowship was awesome and it felt good to go out and not think about how sick I had been feeling. It was good to not have to think about chemo, or Neupogen shots, or having blood work done. It felt good not having to think about having cancer and for a time just being my old-self again. The girls were great and we really need to do more fellowshipping like this in the

future. It felt good being my old self again. I miss who I was before my diagnosis and hadn't realized how my thought process had changed until now. I know things will return to normal and this is just a process and for now I have to deal with it and I trust God through it all. And yes there are times I become a bit anxious because I want it all to end however I don't want to miss the lesson in the process. So for now I will take tonight for the gift it was, thank God for it and continue living in the Season of Anticipation when I know I will be restored, refined and renewed. To God be all the glory!!

Sunday, March 11, 2012
The countdown really begins now. Thirteen more days until my last chemo treatment. This week will be the week I'll have to try my best to steer off the nausea. I have to remember to double up on the anti-nausea medication. Boy! Some of the women in the center that have been under-going chemo for years are really inspirational. I met a woman last week who said she has been going for chemo for about 16 years. Her treatments had been sporadic but when they began they would lust for a few years. You know, I began to realize that my cross that I had been carrying wasn't so bad after-

all these measly 4 months of chemo was nothing compared to what some of these women are going through. Going through chemo for years on a weekly basis is quite taxing on the body, and yes a few women need blood transfusions, had to be hospitalized and oh the hair. For some reason it seemed that they wore their shaved heads with dignity. There was no shame; no fear and nothing shy about their conditions. Their countenance spoke as if to say, "This is me for now, this is what I am going through but I will make it." I have to admit before I started chemo, I was informed during my counseling session that I would lose my hair. It didn't bother me at first but then as I started chemo I began to have reservations. I didn't want to lose my hair and I didn't want to wear a wig. I had braids in my hair so during my treatments I was scared to take them out. Well one day I pulled on one of the braids and it just ripped itself off my scalp. I managed to save the rest of the braid from completely falling off and I made a B-Line to my hair dresser. I was too afraid to take my hair out so she did it for me. I could not believe the amount of hair that came out but my hairdresser worked with my hair and came through for me. Praise God! She was able to re-braid my hair and make it look good in the process. She's the best! It's so funny because after I had my hair done, I went to my doctor's appointment for a follow-up exam and my doctor even noticed I had my hair done. I let him know that I had experienced some hair loss but was still able to have it braided. He thought it was the most amazing thing and told me my hair was resilient. I know I will have to have it cut at some point but for now I'll just make do with what I am able to keep in braids. A nice short hairdo will suffice until my hair regains its strength after the chemo. God, please strengthen me for whatever you have in store for me. You've bought me this far and I know it is your will to see me to the end. I know how I feel about having a bald head but God knows what I will be able to withstand so if it should ever come to that I will just have to bear it. A sistah's gotta do what a sistah's gotta do.

Monday, March 25, 2012
Today is the second day of my church revival and I know that God will truly have a word for us today. Not sure what it is but I am sure it will be better news than what I received on the 22nd of March when I was rushed to the hospital. I had been having upper pain on the left and right side of my back for a few days which began to get

progressively worse. Thinking it was due to a long car drive I had taken that previous weekend and having issues with my back to begin with I went to work as usual. However, during the latter part of the afternoon, the pain became very severe and I began to have shortness of breath. I got up to try and walk it off and my breath grew shorter and shorter. My co-worker told me I had gas so go into the bathroom and let it out but I knew this was more than gas. My supervisor became very worried and wanted to call 911. However, I didn't to be in Taunton without them knowing my medical history so I convinced her to drive my car and take me to Women and Infants. She called my sister who met us there and I was rushed into emergency immediately. After a few questions that I was able to answer between breaths and a shot of morphine for the pain I was able to catch my breath and relax a bit. I was given a C-A-T scan which revealed I had P.E. - Pulmonary Embolisms better known as blood clots in my lungs and I was told I had quite a few of them. The blood was clotting in my lungs and cutting off my circulation. My doctor informed me chemo usually induces clotting of the blood. However, the clot had to have started in my legs and worked its way up. So now I am on Lovenox and Coumadin which are blood thinners. One of which I have to inject myself in the stomach twice a day. And Friday it was supposed to be my last round of chemo so now, they postponed it to the following Friday, however I had been anticipating that day since I began chemo so yes I went crying to my doctor during my follow-up exam after my overnight stay in the hospital and let him know about the delay. He called the supervisor of the chemo center and got me in for that Monday at 9 a.m. Praise God!! I know this is just a test I am going through but God will surely get all the praise, honor and glory through it all.

Tuesday, March 26, 2012
Praise God!! Today was the last day of chem. I was so glad as I was sitting in the room while my treatment was being administered. I began to reflect upon the time I began chemo and all the weeks, (18 of them in all) I had to endure in order to combat this disease. I give God all the praise because He has been my rock through it all. He has had His hand upon me all this time and I must say I felt His presence every step of the way. My sister told me I have been very calm and easy-going through this whole process and if she ever had to go through something such as this she hopes she will be able to have the same

demeanor as I. I just did like Mary did and pondered these things in my heart. I know from whence cometh my help and the only way God will get the glory is by my actions. As I left the doctor's office after my treatment, I felt like I had finished something that God know I would be able to accomplish and endure. Kind of like His challenge to Satan when He said, "Have you considered my servant Job?" I'd like to think God had that same thought as He said, "Have you considered my servant Kathy?" Regardless of anything the enemy may have, I know God will see me through till the end.

Thursday, April 5, 2012
Yesterday I had an appointment with my Surgeon Dr. T. She is all business but very caring and approachable and although I know I am not her only patient, she makes me feel as if I am. She let me know that because of the blood clots in my lungs they will have to postpone my surgery for at least 3 months until they find a way to remove the mass in my breast without causing more clotting during surgery. She said that the clotting threw them for a loop because it was unexpected but they will have to work with it and decide how to approach the situation in the best manner possible. I know regardless of what happened God will get all the

glory and He will have to step in either by a miracle or by showing my doctor the best way to treat his daughter. Everything is in God's hands. My job is to trust and believe. Praise God!

Tuesday, April 24, 2012
Today I had a doctor's appointment with my primary care doctor. I had to get a referral from him to continue my oncology treatments but boy did I get so much more. After speaking with my doctor he began to tell me about what I could expect in regards to the medications I have been taking and the way my other doctors may go about performing my surgery. Then at the end of the conversation he said, "regardless of what happens Kathy just believe that God will bring you through this." I was thrown for a loop because out of all the years I have been going to any doctor, I have never heard one of them mention God. Then he proceeds to tell me that no matter how good the treatment I am getting and no matter how experienced the doctors are, none of them would be able to do their job if it weren't for Christ. I let my doctor know that I pray all the time and that my life is in Christ but that he has encouraged me with his words. My doctor ministered to me with such an anointing that I began to cry in his

office. After my appointment he let me know I would be alright and I left in high spirits. What an awesome appointment.

Thursday, April 26, 2012
Today I had another appointment with Dr. M. She works at a radiation center and she began to explain to me what I can expect if I should need radiation after my surgery. My other doctor, Dr. S has not ruled out more chemo; however radiation is also an option depending on the outcome. It seems like a waiting game now and I just want all this to be done and over with. I thank God for all the strength he has given me to endure this trial because without Him I would be pulling my hair out. God is so awesome. How great thou Art!!!

Thursday, May 24, 2012
So much has happened since the last entry of this journal. I am still on blood thinners and have to have my blood checked every week. I have finally been given a date for my surgery, which is June 1. Yesterday I had a filter surgically implanted to prevent any blood clots from entering my lungs and/or my heart. This is because they will be taking me off my blood thinning medication before my surgery and clotting could occur

anytime during this period. I have to
say that I have been truly blessed
through this whole ordeal. Be it my
family, my church family and especially
the medical staff. God has put
everyone in my path that will make this
a positive journey for me. My eyes
were even more open to this when I was
having my filter put in at Rhode Island
Hospital. The staff was excellent and
there was one nurse who especially made
my day. While they were prepping me
for surgery, the hospital was testing
the electrical system so there was
static on the intercom. It was rather
annoying so the nurse said she was
going to sing for me so I wouldn't have
to hear the static. I didn't take her
seriously so I began to laugh and to my
surprise she began to sing "All Night
Long" by Lionel Richie. Then she began
to dance, (if that's what she calls it)
which made it even funnier. She was so
impressed with herself that she thought
she should try out for "America's Got
Talent." I wanted to advise her not to
do it but considering I was about to
undergo anesthesia I didn't want
anything more done to me than what I
was there for so I kept my mouth shut.
However to my delight, her colleagues
informed her it was not a good idea so
she was satisfied with their critique
and we all had a good laugh in the
process. You know, when I think about

this ordeal I think about Job and I compare myself to what he went through in his body. He had faith through it all and so did I, but one thing he didn't have was laughter. Thank God for the laughter.

Wednesday, June 6, 2012
The surgery on June 1st went well, better than ever the doctors expected. That's the power of the Holy Spirit. My family from Atlanta and New York came up to be with me during and after my surgery and I thank God they were there. Surgery was about 3 hours and my family was told that the doctors believe all traces of cancer were removed. They will know more once the pathology report comes back. I was in the hospital for a day and a half and my sister from Atlanta stayed with me all week. Today I have been given some alone time and found myself crying because I can't even concentrate on my recovery because of being worried about paying bills and other living expenses. Not to mention it all began with me dispensing fluid from a drain that has been placed in my body because of the removal of lymph nodes under my arm. My God, how has it come to this? I am tired and fed up, but I cannot deny the strength that keeps me going. I cannot deny the power of God that sustains me and I certainly cannot deny the

provisions God has made for me and my children. I hate the fact that I trust God for my healing, but worry about my finances. I hate that I trust God to provide good medical care for me but worry about my other household needs. My God, please help me with a complete and total faith makeover. I know God's grace can never be earned, per Romans 11:6 and that faith is the only way to God's grace per Eph 2:8-9 so God please forgive me for my lack of faith for the things that you and you alone already know that I need. God has been so awesome through this whole ordeal I cannot give anyone the praise but Him. And even through my shortcomings and my faults He still remained faithful and committed to His plan for my life. Thank you God for your gift of grace and mercy. It is only by your grace that I will overcome to be more than a conquerer.

Thursday, June 7, 2012
Today I have to go for more blood work for the medication I am taking. The range of motion in my arm has improved a great deal and I have stopped taking the pain medication. Not only because of the pain subsiding but because my heartbeats felt irregular. Especially when I was asleep. I received flowers yesterday from my church family and they were so beautiful. I thank God

for all He has put in my life. I also thank Him for saving and keeping me, especially during a time such as this. I have a hope and a promise. A future that is as bright as can be as long as I keep Christ first. How awesome is that??

Friday, June 8, 2012
Well today I am once again loping around my house because of the limited activity I have been told to do by my doctor. My sister will be going back home to Atlanta tomorrow and although I am grateful for her being here for me I am looking forward to some time to myself. This whole week I have been feeling as if everything and everybody has been so intrusive on my space. It's becoming harder for me to spend the time with God that I am use to spending. I still read my word but there is something that I know I need from God and I am unable to connect right now. Yesterday, I prayed that the Holy Spirit would provide whatever it was that I did not know now or what to ask for. Since the surgery there have been so many emotional psychological changes within me and right now I need serious direction. After surgery, I remember waking up in my room after being in recovery. My family was allowed to visit me and as they were walking in I recall my oldest

Conquerer "My Journey with Cancer"

son James coming over to the bed, leaning over, kissing me on my cheek and whispering in my ear, "you're so strong." I remember telling him that I try and he reassured me that I was. How is it that I do not feel what other people see? I believe the times when I should have been knocked down from chemo, is when God had made me strong. I believe when the doctors thought they were gonna have to do a whole or partial mastectomy and it didn't' really phase me was when I was strong. (By the way they only took out a lump.) I believe being able to continue to work even through chemo, when the doctors were willing to put me out of work, was when God provided the strength. Making it through the operation better than the doctors expected was no one but God telling me I am strong through His provisions. And although I didn't have to say anything, God allowed others to see it, even my son. Thank you God, for your unmerited favor, your grace and mercy upon my life. It is only through you that I have obtained the strength that others see. It is only through you that I have been able to continue to provide for my household and show others that I may have cancer but it doesn't have me. The enemy has infiltrated the wrong camp. His men have been defeated because of the strength of the "one" who abides within. (1 John 4:4) "He who is in you is greater than he who is in the world."

Thursday, June 14, 2012
Today I did a post-op visit with my surgeon. I was anxious for her to remove the drain that I needed after surgery. While waiting in the exam room I began to wonder what the pathology report would be in regards to the results of any cancer being left in my breast. I didn't have to wait very long. When she entered the room she greeted me warmly as usual and asked me how I had been doing since the operation. I told her I had been doing fine but still had some soreness under my arm. She checked the drain and concluded it could be removed and she also removed a few bandages. After another thorough exam she told me she wanted to go over the pathology report. I became really attentive because of the concerned tone in her voice. She informed me that during surgery they discovered more cancerous cells than what was shown on my x-rays. Even before surgery my doctors said this would be a possibility so it was no surprise to me. She also let me know that there were 20 cancerous lymph nodes under my arm and that was way more than they anticipated. The

cancerous tumor in my breast was larger than they thought so they had to move a lot of tissue around and reconstruct the breast in order to accommodate the area that was left empty once the tumor was removed. She went on to tell me that they went through great lengths to remove all of the cancer they could find even going behind the breast, however the pathology report showed that I still have an area of cancer in my breast which means I will have to once again go through chemo. I couldn't believe it. Just when I thought I was getting my life back. Just when I thought I had cleared the hurdle it seems I am back to square one. I am not mad, nor am I sad. Actually I am rather calm about the whole thing. I just thought this was going to be something I could put behind me but I guess not. I know eventually this too shall pass but for now I will continue to always put God first because He bought me through before and He will do it again. I will get more in depth information about my chemo treatments from my primary physicians the following week but when I left the office I had a slew of appointments for genetic testing, physical therapy and follow ups. As I enter the elevator to leave I began to realize I am truly living the 23rd Psalm. Praise God!!

Monday, June 18, 2012
I have had a lot of phone calls over the weekend which was a blessing to me. Words of endearment and encouragement which I truly needed. After receiving the news of my test after the operation, I was asked if I ever thought about getting a full mastectomy. I had thought about it but not in the sense where I would want it for myself. I have encountered women at the doctor's office that had no choice but to have their breast removed and even then I found it unsettling. I am not in the place right now where I am willing to have a part of my body totally removed regardless of the circumstances. Yes it can be reconstructed but right now I don't feel led to do anything drastic such as that. I have stopped sharing what I am going through with some people because they tend to put you in a space that is not your own. They become very opinionated and make me feel as if what I am doing is wrong because it wouldn't be what they would do. I believe if God wanted my breast to be removed He would not have allowed me to catch the cancer in time. I thank God I haven't told too many people, because right now I don't need opinions I need prayer for strength, guidance, faith and direction and my compass, Jesus Christ has and never will mislead me.

Thursday, June 20, 2012
Today I visited Dr. S for a follow-up appointment. I could tell there was something pressing on his mind when he entered the room so I decided to break the ice and compliment him on his attire. He wore a sage green shirt with matching pants but a little darker. I could tell he was a little embarrassed by the compliment but flattered nonetheless. Besides, this was not my first time complimenting him on his clothes so I'm sure he is a little use to it. I usually tease him about his administrative abilities whenever I give him paperwork that needs to be filled out. This day was no different. I've come to realize that I have been more accepting of what God has given me strength to endure than some of the medical staff at the medical center. So when they show signs of upset and unrest I use tactics and ice breakers to let them know that regardless of the prognosis I will be alright. After my examination, Dr. S pulled up a chair and began to go through my chart with me. He informed me of the total removal of the cancerous tumor however; when a sample of the tissue that was taken after surgery was examined at the lab it came back positive for active cancerous cells. Although the cells had not fully developed into cancer, there

still a possibility that it could turn into full blown cancer again. What made it even worse was that it just wasn't a few cells; it was particles all over and within my breast. I sat there pretty stunned but not alarmed. My whole attitude was, o.k. what do, we do next. I just want to keep it moving to the next phase. Dr. S informed me I would have to undergo more chemo but it will be every two weeks. This phase of chemo will be much stronger than the first doses I was getting before surgery and I will be given anti-nausea medication that will last for three days. He let me know about the side effects and was still amazed that I was still able to get my hair braided. He gave me a prescription for more nausea meds and I was also given a prescription to Ruth's for special undergarments. As I made my appointment for my first chemo treatment which was June 28, 2012 I was granted my special request to have the same nurse I had before, Sandra. The nurse with the smiling eyes.

Friday, June 21, 2012
Today I began physical therapy with Dr. G. He is a very gentle man in stature with freckles, huge hands and a strong accident. He taught me how to massage my arm and how to begin the flow of fluids in my upper body toward my arm.

I am loving the ambience of the room, mainly because I have never been to a physical therapist. I am also loving a lamp in the corner of the room that would fit perfectly in my living room or dining room. Every time the doctor leaves the room I run over to the lamp to see who the manufacturer was so I can look them up online.

After my session, I am a bit sore but feeling good nonetheless. He tells me to continue my therapy at home until our next session, but I know I won't. Maybe every now and then I will do stretching exercises but that's it. I leave my therapist feeling good really wanting to go back to work. Staying at home is the pits but I know my health is more important right now. Besides, Dr. S doesn't want to release me until after my chemo treatments. Well, I'll see how I do on these treatments and if I get through it I'm gonna ask to go back to work. I just like feeling productive.

Thursday, June 28, 2012
Today I am beginning my second round of chemo. I am here in the late afternoon and it is pretty crowded. I am happy to see all of the nurses and some of the patients who are familiar to me regardless of the circumstances. I praise God for the high spirits I am in

as I sit here getting my anti-nausea meds administered intravenously. Earlier I had physical therapy and I saw my nurse Sandy. I truly missed her warm spirit and smiling eyes as she greeted me before my therapy session. She informed me after noticing I still had my braids that the type of chemo I was going to be getting was a lot stronger than the other chemo I was getting. I later found out the stronger the chemo called "Adriamyan" or red devil as it is called is a type of chemo that has to be manually administered by the nurse for 20 minutes. They call it red devil because the toxins are released via the urine which turns red. When my nurse told me that before I leave I would be peeing red urine I thought she was joking but she informed me she wasn't. So now I have the attitude of "Boy I can't wait to see this." The other drug she told me about was Cytoxan. She let me know I would feel sinus pressure with this drug but that should be the only side effect. I am so not looking forward to losing my hair but I know I have to eventually face reality. I have already bought some scarves for my hair; however I am not mentally ready yet. I guess God is not through with removing all the layers of yucky stuff that is separating me from Him. Maybe there are things He still wants me to let go of so more of me can depend on Him and not on other sources. God has proven himself time and time again that He will never leave me nor forsake me. He will always supply my needs and He will never fail me. And He hasn't. And because of this, I will face my reality and if I should lose my hair, so be it. I will just have to wear a scarf and look good in it too. Nearly every woman in here is wearing a bald head and not even caring. To them it is what it is!! I'll have to adapt to that attitude. Vanity is truly something isn't it? Wasn't that one of Satan's traits? Wasn't pride another one of his downfalls? Okay God, if those layers are vanity and pride, remove them ASAP and please forgive me for even making them a part of my walk with you. Okay one of my meds is almost finished so I have to begin the second part of this entry later. To God be all the glory.

<u>Saturday, July 7, 2012</u>
Today is the first day I feel a little normal after receiving chemo once again. I have been sick for eight and a half days and I am so tired of this right now. I was sick on my birthday and on the fourth of July as well. God please take this awful feeling away. This is truly no way for anyone to live. I am going to ask my doctor

about the dosage he is giving me because I don't think nausea should last this long. I can't really eat anything because I don't know what will affect me afterwards so I just eat fruits, which I love anyway, I try to eat meat but I have to watch the vegetables because certain ones will interact negatively with my blood thinning medication. I have become irritable, withdrawn and frustrated. The only reason I answer the phone is because I know people are calling because they care and are praying for me. My aunt advised me to buy the wristbands people wear on the cruises to stop the nausea and I thought that was a good idea. I bought them and it did subside a bit but my stomach cannot take mild products too well. I miss being in church but to drive in my car or anyone else's is not too appealing. I can't drive my car because I am too sick and I don't want to drive in anyone else's car because then I will be pulled into having a conversation when all I want to do is just crawl up somewhere and forget about everything. I wake up and the first thing on my mind is "another day dealing with being sick." I ask God to forgive me when this happens because I realize it's not about me it's about Him and always has been. It is so easy to lose your way when a constant distraction, a thorn in your side is always there. Well, today is a new day and I will use it wisely. Thank you God for today...

Monday, July 17, 2012
Today I have discovered my hair is falling out. Not shedding here and there but falling out at the roots. I am literally picking my hair out of my scalp and it is freaking me out. I didn't experience this type of hair loss the first time I began chemo so I was able to wear my hair in braids, but with this new type of chemo my hair began to fall out after the second treatment. Boy o'boy is this a test or what? I tell ya, God is good through it all and now I have to really take my faith up a notch and get through this hurdle as well. Not that taking my faith up a notch is something that seems like a chore; however I am still in the midst of the realm of all that is going on in my body. So I guess taking my faith up a notch is not a bad thing after all. I saw my doctor in passing when I went for blood work and he asked me how I was doing. I informed him I was doing okay but that now my hair is falling. He told me he understood but to look at the bright side. My hair would grow back and his wouldn't. We had a good laugh on the elevator, said good-bye in the lobby

and parted ways. Well, head-wraps and wigs here I come…

Sunday, July 22, 2012
Today I finally did it! I had the rest of my hair shaved off. I am still getting use to it and I thank God I have a round shapely head. I kept some of the hair and had some pictures taken for keepsake. My aunt showed me a new way to sport my new do with a make-up session and I must say she did a great job. It's very airish up there even in the heat. So I keep a head wrap on but slowly I am trying to get use to this new do. I'm not sure if I ever will, not sure if I want to. Am I being taken out of my comfort zone? Is this the layer of vanity God is trying to remove from me? Work with me Lord because only you know I am not willing to take on this new appearance head on. I need to pass this test so I can get to the next level in Christ Jesus. I've learned that if I stay at the same level in Christ Jesus for more than one day I have back-slidden. Every day should be a growing process no matter how small the progression. Lord, forgive me for back-sliding and help me to not focus on my appearance but to focus on you and the glory you so deserve through all of this…

Monday, August 6, 2012
Last week was an awesome week for me. After my third round of chemo I was expecting to feel sick as usual but to my delight I didn't' feel sick at all. The whole week was great and I thank God because I know it was nobody but Him. He showed me what to eat to keep the nausea away and as I obeyed my days got better and better. I was even able to make it to church on Sunday and it felt awesome to be there. My church family is the best. It felt great being with them again and the well wishes and love I felt was more than I could bear. I know they are praying for me because I feel their prayers in the mast of my recovery. I have another round of chemo this Thursday and that will be it. I thank and praise God for all He has done and will continue to do in my life.

Tuesday, August 7, 2012
Yesterday I went to a workshop at the Breast Health Center. The workshop was given by a group of hairdressers who wanted to help the patients feel comfortable with the treatments they were going through. Everyone had lost their hair so this was a great opportunity for us to learn about make-up and how to wear certain head-wraps to make us more secure in our temporary setback. Upon my arrival, it seemed

everyone had already settled in and was applying make-up or making small talk. I sat next to a young girl who still had all of her hair and was wondering how far into her treatment she was I knew when I first began chemo in November of 2011 I never lost my hair so I wondered if she had the same type of chemo as I did. As the workshop progressed I learned how to apply make-up and how to wear head-wraps in different styles and sat in wonderment at how helpful all this information was to me. Not to mention the care and support we received from the hairdressers. At the end of the workshop we sat around for a bit and began to chat and by that time I had become familiar with the young lady sitting next to me so I asked her if she had been coming to the center long and she shook her head no and began to cry. My heart went out to her and I began to reassure her that everything would be okay. She began to tell me that she had only been coming to the center for a week but that everyone had been so nice. She continued to share that it had been a whirlwind with all of the appointments she has been having and all of the test she has had to endure and that she was concerned because she had two small children ages 5 years and 1 year old. My heart really went out to her and I shared with her that she was in the best of care and from the information we received from the workshop God had already put everything in order for her because the resources were in her neighborhood. Once everyone heard me mention God they were all over it. They too began to let her know that God will take care of her and because she was having surgery that following week we all let her know she would be in our prayers. We all gave her a hug as she was leaving and as I walked out the door into the hallway one of the hairdressers said, "Once you mentioned God we were all over it." I smiled at her and thanked her for her time and as I walked to the elevator I realized this is the type of society we live in. We cannot mention God because of who we might offend. Believe me, after my experience with cancer all the appointments, tests, chemo, surgeries, implants and medications there would be no-way I would want to go through this by myself. People cannot be there for you all the time and sometime you don't want anyone around but God. I know God will be there for that young lady and her family just like He has been there for me and my family and for all the other patients and their families as well.

Thursday, August 9, 2012

Okay so I am truly bummed out today. I arrive at my appointment for my last chemo treatment only to find out it will not be administered because I have a fever of 101.8. I really was looking forward to getting this over with. God knows how much I hate this new chemo drug they are giving me. Now I have to wait a whole week to finalize this treatment. I arrive home feeling disappointed but accepting what has happened and began working on this fever that I realize is starting to progress. I'll take an Ibuprofen to see what happens…

Friday, August 18, 2012

Well, the Ibuprofen worked. I sweat the fever out all night long even with the air blowing on me. However, later in the afternoon it was back to square one. I had another fever of 102 and the chills were awful. What in the world is going on? Not to mention I am becoming short of breath very easily. I refuse another stay in the hospital so Lord, take control of these white blood cells and get rid of whatever is causing these chills and fever. Thank you Lord; because I know it's already done.

Conquerer "My Journey with Cancer"

Monday, August 20, 2012 (10:02 a.m.)
Today is the last day of my chemo treatments. My appointment is at 1:30 p.m. however I have to be examined by a nurse to make sure I can have this last treatment. I know I will be able to so I am already praising God.

Monday, August 20, 2012 (2:47 p.m.)
Okay I am sitting at my last chemo session and glory to God I have been given a clean bill of health. My doctor's assistant let me know that I have been really strong through it all and that I have come a long way. I will still have to come here but not for chemo and it will be once every three weeks. I am sitting next to a woman who says she has been battling ovarian cancer for four years. She said they only gave her three years to live but her and I agreed that her final days are in the hands of God. It's very comforting to talk with the staff and patients of the Breast Center because the majority of them believe and have their faith in God. Thank you God for being in the midst of everything and in everyone.

Tuesday, August 21, 2012
Today I realized I did not commemorate the anniversary of my first entry. It was August 17, 2011 and that was the first day I discovered the tumor in my

breast. It has been a long journey since that day. A journey filled with good days, bad days, laughter, tears, frustration and sometimes confusion. So many tests, appointments, illnesses, hospital stays and the medications are unbelievable. When I think back I can only thank God for all the strength he has provided. Even on days when I just wanted to throw in the towel. You're awesome God!! What a friend I have in You.

Tuesday, August 28, 2012
Early this morning about 2 a.m. I woke up on my couch after a defeated attempt to watch television. I lay there for a while and decide to get up and turn my son's T.V. off in his room before getting into my own bed. Well I stand up and begin to walk to his room feeling just fine when all of a sudden I see blackness and I pass out. I come to as I am falling up against a chair and slam onto the floor. My son jumps up scared out of his sleep and wits and asking what was that. He realizes it was me and comes to help. I lay back on the couch a little shaken from the ordeal and not really knowing what happened. I was fine until passing out. It seemed as if everything had been lifted out of me and my body just fell. Psalms 39:4 states "let me know how fleeting is my life." Truly I had

no control over what happened. There was nothing for me to fight off, nothing I could prevent from happening. God had all things in His hands. As I lay on the couch pondering all this I begin to laugh because once I became aware of my son jumping up out of his sleep I realized it was the funniest thing at that moment. I try not to let him see me laugh because I know he was scared and concerned so I will let him calm down for now and let him know about the comedic side to all of this in the morning. I thank God for showing me the lighter side of things even in the midst of all that I am going through. Thank you God for the gift of laughter.

Wednesday, August 29, 2012
Today is the day I was to have my filter removed. It was placed to stop any blood clots during my surgery and now it is time to take it out. I am prepared for this minor and quick surgery and I am wheeled into the operating room. I am brief on what to expect before and after and then everyone begins to prepare for surgery. All of a sudden I am told I will be feeling some stinging and pressure to which I thought would be no big deal since they had not yet anesthised me. However, to my dismay I am feeling them cut into my neck and inserting the

instrument to remove the filter. Now I did not feel this when they inserted the filter so what has changed since? O.K. now that the pain is over they are viewing the filter only to realize they cannot remove it because there is a large blood clot inside the filter. O.M.G.!! However the good news is that it was a good thing the filter was there because only God knows what the outcome would have been. Yes, God only knows about the outcome that is why He planned to have the filter put in my body to begin with. SO I am sent back home with instructions from my doctor to increase my blood thinning medication in hopes that the blood clot will dissolve itself. As I leave the hospital I thank God for watching over me and for the filter blocking the blood clot, then in typical me fashion I become angry because I was told to fast before surgery and it was all for nothing and now I am starving. I have always been a breakfast person but I had to nauseous in the morning for a surgery that never even took place. Yes there was an attempt by the recovery room staff to give me luck consisting of a dry turkey sandwich, 2 cranberry drinks; peaches and a package of gold fish. O.M.G.!! Will the real plate of food stand up please!!! My sister took me to the cafeteria and bought me a pizza with pepperoni and a diet Coke. However while eating; I am having visions of fried chicken, mac and cheese with yellow rice dancing through my head. I cannot get to the grocery store fast enough. Praise God!!

Journal 2

Thursday, September 6, 2012
Yesterday I had an appointment with my doctor. He informed me that I had a normal echocardiogram so my heart was strong enough to begin my radiation treatments. He also informed that I had low white and red blood cells. Now a few days prior I was in the emergency room because I had fainted and was easily short of breath. I was given an option of whether or not to have a blood transfusion after my lab results returned and I chose not have it; however my doctor said he wanted me to have the transfusion because my red cells needed to be at a certain level before starting radiation. He ordered more blood work before I left the office to see if there were any improvements in my blood count since my visit to the emergency room. I left the visit feeling very upset about the transfusion and not wanting to go through with it. My doctor asked me if it was for religious reasons as to why I didn't want the transfusion and I

told him "no." I just didn't want to get rid of one disease just to contract another. He assured me the procedure of screening candidates that give blood and the testing of blood is very rigorous and safe and is not the way it used to be. I arrived home feeling very uneasy about the whole thing. I want to call my doctor and tell him forget about it and I am not doing it, but I began to think about how far I have come and to stop or hinder my recovery now will be a waste of everything I have been through. As I am logging in this journal I receive a call from my doctor's office telling me that my blood level is improving and that I may not need the transfusion, but they will speak with the radiation office to see what they want to do. As I wait for the phone call I pray extra hard that I will not need the transfusion but the return phone call did not work in my favor. I will need one unit of blood to begin radiation. Right now I feel as if everything is coming against me. I am beginning to feel very irritated with the smallest thing and I just want to be normal again. I'm tired of it all. I'm tired of crying, I'm tired of having to be strong when I wish someone was here to be strong for me. I have had people say I inspire them. Boy, I wish I felt that inspiration. I know God is working everything out on my behalf but sometimes I feel I just can't win. I know this too shall pass but being in the midst of it right now makes seeing the finish line difficult. I know when people read or hear this that they will have their own opinions and scriptures to make me feel victorious or to tell me that God has never left my side. Well let me tell you, I already know that!! I already know about God's healing power, His grace and His mercy. But until you walk in my shoes, until you are hooked up to a chemo machine with a substance being pumped into your body that causes you to be ill for days on end, until you have to make numerous trips to the emergency room because your red and white blood cells have dropped to a critical level, until you have been admitted into the hospital because the blood in your lungs is clotting and cutting off your air supply, until you are so fatigued that you are unable to enjoy life the way you used to or until your hair falls out along with your eyebrows and eyelashes, then you can come to me and tell me your secret of always being happy and jovial. As my pastors always say, "If you have never been attacked by the enemy and you are always happy, sit down and get saved." I am glad to know that I am good and saved because through this whole ordeal I have not always been a happy camper. But God's strength has been made perfect in my weakness. I have allowed myself to feel the emotions as they come, but I have also allowed the Holy Spirit to deal with situation in due time. I thank God for allowing me to be the human being that I am and for making room for me to express my feelings and emotions because after my crying fits and tantrums, He graciously shows me His love by comforting me and showing me a more excellent way.

Friday, September 7, 2012
Today I had the blood transfusion and felt really "icky" inside. I know the transfusions saves lives and I am not trying to downplay this procedure at all but this is how I am feeling when it comes to me and my situation at this moment. While sitting in the waiting area, I began to cry just knowing I had to do this and that there was no alternative. I'm glad the other patient in the waiting area had her back to me as she watched television so I felt a bit of privacy was granted for me to shed a few tears. I received calls and well wishes from my family letting me know they loved me and that they are praying for me. I wipe my eyes just in time as my nurse; Sandra calls me into the room. She knows how I feel about getting this procedure so

she has a concerned look on her face coupled with a smile that reaches her eyes. I know her intentions were to put me at ease so I try to pull myself together. She gives me Ibuprofen and Benadryl and begins the I.V. when the unit of blood is delivered, I automatically knew because it was packed in a "red" cooler. After my nurse administered the blood into the I.V., I watched as it slowly made its way through the tube and into my system. I felt a sense of nausea just knowing that someone else's life blood was flowing through my body. It's funny because before my nurse hooked the blood up to the I.V., I just stared at the unit of blood wondering about the donor and thinking to myself that they donated this blood out of love and here I am not wanting it. They made a sacrifice of themselves and here I am looking down at it. Wow! Sound like something that happened over 2000 years ago doesn't it? Jesus sacrificed his blood only for people to reject it. Well, I began to feel the results of the Benadryl and dozed off. I didn't want to look at that red tube any longer. I was awakened by my nurse to take my vital signs and was also given a pillow to rest my head more comfortably. The whole procedure took about 4 hours and I was glad it was all over. I was given an appointment to return the following Friday to begin my Herceptin treatments. This treatment will stop the growth of cancer cells and will be given to me every third week for about 12-14 treatments. I also begin radiation every day for six weeks. Boy is my body going through! Thank you God for your strength. Don't know what I would do without it.

Monday, September 10, 2012
Yesterday I went to church and was warmly greeted as usual. I try to make as many services as possible when I am feeling well because my body seems to have taken on a life of its own and tends to shut down at times. Rev. Ray spoke about being Luke warm for Christ and he came from Rev. 3:14-22. Through the whole message, I examined my own walk with Christ and compared my walk to when I first began to serve Him until now. I realized I still desire to serve my Lord and Savior but that fiery zeal was not there as it was in the beginning. Could this be because life has gotten in the way? In the beginning I didn't let anything stop me from leaning and growing in Christ. What happened? Is it people I have allowed in my life that I should have left alone? Whatever it is Lord, please remove them or it because I want that zeal that I once had. Yes, I still pray, I still read His word

"EVERY" morning and I still acknowledge Him when speaking to others, but there is just that something that I miss that I had when I first came to Him. The gap that is separating me from Christ is because of me because He has never left His post. Lord, show me the way back so I may close the gap and please not leave me until I am back at your side once again.

Friday, September 14, 2012
Today I received my first dose of Herceptin. This drug is just a preventative measure against the cancer growing. I will be receiving this treatment every 3 weeks for a year. During the treatment I met a nice woman who was getting chemo for the first time. She was receiving the same type of medication called Carboplatin which is what I received when I first began my chemo treatments. We talked for the entire time I was there, however her stay was a little longer. She too was getting her treatments every three weeks so we both were hoping we would be scheduled for the same time. As I was leaving the clinic I realized I didn't get her name nor did I give her my name but I am sure we will see each other again. I find that every woman I encounter at the Breast Center has a very interesting story and I am sure they feel the same when I share my

story with them. It makes the recovery more bearable to know that someone can relate to you and all the different stages it takes to reach if some of them reach it at all. There are stores I have heard of women battling cancer for years then going into remission only to have it resurface. God please cure us all of this dreadful disease.

Thursday, September 20, 2012
Today I received a phone call from one of my sisters in my church apologizing for not being as available to me as she would like. She explained to me that was why she would send me cards, to remind me that she was always thinking about me. She proceeds to tell me that she was also upset with me. I ask her why and she asks me why I didn't tell her about my medical running out. I was taken aback because I hadn't a clue as to what she was talking about, so I asked her, "what are you talking about?" She tells me that it was something she overheard while at bible study the night before. (Sounds like she was eavesdropping). I told her that my medical did not run out and that I only have a co-pay. She says she was just making sure everything was okay however I was curious as to why anyone would be talking about my medical expenses in church. I have never mentioned anything to anyone so where

did the conversation come from and from whom? Well, upon speaking with someone else who was there that night, she began to tell me that there was a raffle being given to certain people in the church on my behalf. Well I knew that was all about because a few weeks ago I learned my union rep was organizing a softball benefit on my behalf. They usually do this for people within our union that are seriously ill or have been through a life altering hardship. Well upon my finding out about the raffles being disbursed, I look at the raffles I had and lo and behold it says that the proceeds will benefit Kathy Brown. Could that have been why she thought I was losing my medical? Usually, when people say the word "benefits," they are talking about medical so maybe that sparked her curiosity. In any event, I know she meant well, however if I was losing my benefits I am not sure how telling her would help me.
Nevertheless, considering the type of person this sister is I know she would have found a way to help me out.
That's just the type of heart she has. May God continue to bless her always…

Friday, September 21, 2012
Today is my son Tevin's birthday. He is 14 years old, 6 ft. tall and wears a size 13 shoe. I thank God for my boys

although parenting is not easy. After a morning of wishing him a happy birthday and dropping him and my other son James off at their respective destinations, I keep my weekly appointment to have blood work done. Afterwards, I high-tail it across town just in time to keep another appointment for a referral from my primary doctor Dr. E.M. Once I in the room my vitals are taken and he walks in and greets me. He remembers me and asks me how I am doing? I say I am fine and he automatically asks me how is my faith. I tell him my faith is all I have and he says good. It is always a pleasure to visit with him because he is the only doctor I have that shares his faith and doesn't mind talking about it. I let him know about the referral and he asks me questions regarding my condition since the last time I was in his office. I let him know about the surgery and the chemo I had afterwards and that now I have to go for radiation. He sat down across from me and began to enter my information into the computer then stopped and looked at me with sincerity in his eyes. He asks if he could share something with me and I said "sure." He began to tell me that the other day he was reading the book of Ezekiel and that it was the only book that talks about the likeness of God. He said

God's presence can only be compared to something we know but it is far greater than what our mind are able to comprehend. He continues to tell me that he was reading about how Ezekiel saw the sky, the ear and saw the firmament (horizon) and when he focused on the firmament he became confused because he saw things that he did not understand but when he looked above the firmament he saw Jesus Christ on the thrown and everything was alright because his focus was now on Jesus and not the firmament which caused confusion and allowed him to not focus on who was in charge. After telling me this, Dr. M told me to not look at the firmament, but look above it and keep my focus on the one who is sitting on the throne. He said as long as I continue to think about things that worry me, make me sad or concentrate on things I don't understand, I will not be able to get direction from Jesus who is always willing to guide me. I was so floored that my doctor would share that with me because for the past few days it was not my health I had been concerned about. I had been concentrating on how I was going to pay my rent while only getting paid half of my paycheck. This has never been a concern of mine because I have always worked but now here I am, battling cancer, out on disability, worried about my rent with one week to go before it is due and no money insight and what does God do? He makes a way for me to have to visit my doctor and tells me to stop looking at the firmament and concentrate on the one who sits above it and who will provide in the words of Smith Wigglesworth, "God is more eager to Answer than we are to ask."

Saturday, September 22, 2012
Yesterday my union representative organized a benefit to assist me in my financial situation. It gets tough when you are trying to maintain your finances on half of what would have been getting if you were working. The event was held at a ballpark in Taunton. So my two sons, my sister and I went and boy did we enjoy ourselves. There was a softball game being played, food raffles, drinks being served, music, karaoke, and a whole lot of socializing. I saw my coworkers for the first time in 3 months and it was so good to see them. My supervisor was there with her awesome new hairdo. She let her hair grow then had it cut and donated her hair to locks of love. An organization that uses human hair to make wigs for cancer patients. The whole day was such a blessing and I couldn't get over the turnout. Even employees from other companies came out

Conquerer "My Journey with Cancer"

to support, such as Budweiser and Home Plate, an Italian restaurant that Verizon Wireless always orders from for lunch and dinner. They even came to feed us while we were on the picket-line. I let them know how much I appreciated all that they have done but for some reason I felt thank you was not enough. To know that people who don't really know me and even those who do would take their time and plan something like this for me is totally beyond what I expected. I enjoyed getting their cards in the mail but this totally blew me away. I thank God for the wonderful time I had and my prayer is that God will bless and protect each and every person that took the time out to care enough to make this event a success whether they were there or behind the scene. I truly work with a bunch of awesome people...God bless them all!!

Tuesday, September 25, 2012
Yesterday was the first day of my radiation treatments. It went well but was really not what I expected. I didn't feel anything just saw beams of light so I guess that was the radiation. The two attendants there were very nice. However, the eldest of the attendants informed her colleague that she was having a mental block and forgot how to prep me for the

treatment. "Hey, no mental blocks on my watch," I thought. Take out a manual, school notes or something but there is no room for error here. To my delights her colleague came to the rescue and all went well. I have 35 more sessions to go and then I will be finished with this part of my post-surgery treatments. Can't wait for the testimony Lord, It's gonna be a good one!

Wednesday, September 26, 2012
Tonight I have another radiation treatment. I was given medication to rub on the area being treated. So as to keep the skin moistened. Last night as I was sitting in the exam room with my doctor, she informed me of how they position the breast to treat it with the radiation. She let me know that because of the severity of my scoliosis, they have to position me differently than others because my heart is closer to my right side than my left. I was taken aback because I never knew that nor was I ever told. I was diagnosed with Scoliosis, which is a curvature of the spine when I was about 10 years old. As I got older, the condition became worse and by the time I had surgery at the age of 13 years old I had an 84 degree curve in my spine. It was corrected to about a 42 degree curve out still the damage is

noticeable. Sometimes when I look in the mirror at myself I wonder why I am made the way I am. Why is my body different that other people? I know the Bible says I am fearfully and wonderfully made but sometimes I don't feel that I look so wonderful. Especially now that I have been diagnosed with cancer, my body has gone through a lot including me losing my hair which I have not gotten use to yet. I look in the mirror and study myself and my journeys and wonder what has happened and where have I gone. Who am I now and what am I supposed to do with this new person staring back at me. People say that I will be an inspiration for others but sometimes I wonder how when I don't even like what I see. I can't even inspire myself to accept this person in the mirror. So how am I going to help someone else? I guess it's all in God's hands to show and guide me in the way I am lost and confused so please Lord help me before it's too late…

Thursday, September 27, 2012
I am currently sitting in Chili's, one of my favorite places to eat. I ordered a BLT and a salad and was going to order another dish to go but thought better of it and declined despite the urging of the waitress. I have come to realize I am an emotional eater. So I

am trying to curb myself when I realize I am only eating because of a certain situation. One of the situations being my finances. I have already gone before God about that and he has sent reinforcements my way in the form of confirmation from other people so I am just waiting for Him to move on my behalf. However, another emotion has surfaced and I have yet to deal with that one. Not that I really have to but old feelings have surfaced regarding a passion of mine that has been put on hold since my diagnosis. Today I had to retrieve my transcript from the university I attended. I have a passion for travel and tourism. So this school was perfect. Not to mention my employer picked up the tab. To make a long story short, while I had been attending school, I loved every single minute of it. The classes, the instructors, the students, everything. When I was diagnosed I had to stop attending after going for about 2 ½ years, so when I went to get my transcript all the old familiar feelings re-surfaced and I realized there had also been a part of me that I missed. That part was the student. The joy of learning about a passion of mine was truly missed and being in the midst of the other students as they made their way to class or Starbucks bought a longing in me that I really didn't think was all that bad. I miss the projects, the smell of the culinary students meals as dinner was being prepared for the other students, the smell of coffee from the other Continuing Education Students that I had class with. Boy O' boy so much is passing me by. But I know so much more is yet to come. Thank you God for what you have done for me, for what you are doing, for what you have yet to do. I know my best interest is all you have in mind.

Wednesday, October 3, 2012
Yesterday was not a good day for me. I was extremely irritated because of my financial situation and it seemed as if everything was closing in on me. I know God would supply for my needs but I just couldn't shake this uneasy feeling of when I would see it or when He was going to do it. This past Sunday, Dec. Jay spoke about how slowly we move when God tells us to do something, but when we want Him to move on our behalf we want Him to move immediately if not sooner. That was where I was yesterday. I wanted something to be done and I wanted it done now!! Even the technicians at the clinic where I get my radiation were irritating me. I have learned not to let my anger or frustration show in certain situations and I must say I did

a pretty good job at it yesterday but I pray I can continue to do so. After my treatments I came home and had to make a few phone calls that I didn't want to make but I had to swallow my pride which I know is one of the worse things God would want me to have because it was one of Satan's traits. To my surprise, after making the phone calls to straighten out my finances everything went well. I'm still clearing up a few things but it is not as bad as it was. Lord, forgive me for the many times I have worried about things you have already told me you would take care of. I have been saved for 17 years and I still do not have the faith I should have in you. Please have mercy on me; this worrying has got to stop in the name of Jesus!

Saturday, October 6, 2012
Last night my granddaughter came over and I was more than happy to see her. I hadn't seen her in a while due to circumstances beyond my control. Nevertheless, it was great to see her. We talked and watched television, cartoons are on all the time when comes over, especially SpongeBob, and she would help me put my head scarf on when I would try to put it on myself. She asked me what had happened to my hair and I told her I had to cut it off because I was sick. It didn't seem to

faze her so I asked her if I could have some of her hair and she was more than willing to give it to me. The innocence and charity of a child is amazing!!

<u>Monday, October 22, 2012</u>
So much has happened since my last entry and I will try to sum it all real briefly because I have a radiation appointment in ½ hour. My bills had been piling up really bad so God has stepped in mightily and took care of that. He has even made a way for me to pay my rent months in advance. The monies from the benefit that was held on my behalf came through and it was a really sizeable amount. That helped me to be able to pay off some other bills and to pay down on others. My hair is really starting to come in now, it's more than just "peach fuzz" so I am happy about that. I participated in my very first "Breast Cancer" walk yesterday and I really enjoyed myself. The encouragement and representation of the participants was overwhelming. I was greatly sore after the walk but still felt good in my heart nonetheless. I will be finished with my radiation soon so I am really excited about that. God is truly moving and I am so excited at what He is doing and is yet to do.

Monday, October 29, 2012

I have been having an awesome week. God has truly been moving on my behalf and for that I am grateful. It's as if I am being rewarded for something out I don't know for what. However, God is like that. He will bless us even if we don't deserve it. Sometimes I am taken aback at how much He loves us. I tend to feel so unworthy of all the blessings He gives to me and to just say, "thank you," does not feel as if it is enough to give back to Him. His blessings outweigh my sins and for that I am forever grateful. I am also grateful for my church family. I know it was no one but my Savior that has planted me at GTOM because I would not have known how to pray to be amongst such people during my walk with Christ. All the prayers, the well wishes, the hugs and love that I have been blessed to receive during my struggle is beyond measure. I can honestly say that my church is filled with the love of God. I cannot imagine, nor would I want to be anywhere else but at my home church for the things I need from God. I know there are people that are truly praying for me and I thank God for that. May God continue to bless and keep GTOM forevermore if not longer.

Wednesday, October 31, 2012
Today is Halloween and everyone is still digging themselves out of a storm that we had a day and a half ago. Hurricane Sandy will surely go down in history as one of the worst storms ever. Especially for New York. I was talking with my aunt and she informed me that 1/3 of New York is without power. She said the city that never sleeps has finally gone to sleep. There were a few people that expressed to me their concerns about the storm but for some reason or another I was not concerned at all. I obviously prepared myself for what may happen but the overall concern was not there. I began to ask myself why there was a lack of concern, why I felt as if this hurricane was just a rainy day and I came to the conclusion that Sandy was a storm that other people were going through. It was not my storm. My storm began over a year ago and although it was not a raging storm anymore, the clean-up continues. Hurricane Sand was a Category One. My storm was grade 3 cancer and disaster relief is still on the scene. My prayers are with those who have lost loved ones, homes and possessions and one day I know they will rise above their current situation stronger and wiser. I too will rise above my current situation stronger, wiser and

above all else, closer to God. Yesterday, as I was leaving my radiation appointment, I walked into the foyer of the doctor's office to see the sun peeking through the clouds as if it assured us that a brighter day was near. I walked to my car and all the while knowing that God has a plan for the sun to rise on my situation. There are days where it peeks thru the clouds, but I know a full viewing of the sun is near and just knowing God has that for me is truly a blessing. Praise His Holy Name!!!

Monday, November 4, 2012
This weekend I attended my church's annual women's ministry breakfast at Venies De Milo restaurant. What an awesome time in the Lord we had. It was good to sit down with everyone in a setting that didn't require us to do anything but socialize and enjoy the company of one another. Evangelist Ruby was the speaker and I truly enjoyed her analogy of how the birds that fly south are all on one accord while trying to reach their destination. She compared their flight with the body of Christ. The birds are on one mind and one accord and they are following the leader of the squad. If there is a bird that is sickly and cannot make the trip these are two birds will land with the sickly bird

and tend to his needs. This should be the plight of the church and I must say, since my diagnosis I have had more than one person tending to my needs in the church. My brothers and sisters in the Lord have been awesome and to just say "Thank You," does not seem to be enough. As I sat at the breakfast I began to look around and was touched by all the women that came out. I began to realize that we all have a story to tell that would help someone else just like those birds help each other. I pray that with all I am enduring, my story will be able to help someone to persevere and press forward while keeping God their main source of strength. I was one of those birds, flying to a destination when all of a sudden I became ill. God sent people to tend to me until I am able to join the flock again and continue my journey. I am beginning to once again regain my position slowly but surely and I cannot wait until I am once again flying high with the healing power of Jesus Christ in my wings. I have noticed that when the birds fly South, they fly in a "V" formation. This enables them to help the other birds behind them fly much easier in order to bear the long journey. I believe for the body of Christ we must form a "V" formation for victory because when a brother or sister is down and is raised back up the devil is defeated and the power of God is shown victorious. What could be better than that?"? Amen...

<u>Wednesday, November 7, 2012</u>
This morning I am in good springs because Obama has been re-elected as President. It has been a very combative election year between Obama and Romney but in the end the people spoke loud and clear. All day I tried not to look at the results but I just couldn't help it. I fell asleep on my couch last night after talking with a friend of mine about the election. We both didn't want to wake up disappointed. So we kept switching between channels to see who would win Ohio which is the state that would really decide the winner. I fell asleep only to be awakened by my friend calling me and saying that Obama had won Ohio. I jumped off my couch and began thanking and praising God. Not to mention I prayed over my ballot when I was resting. God is good!! After I left the poles on yesterday, I went to get my weekly blood work done then I went to my daily radiation appointment. As I sat in the waiting area, another patient and I began to talk about how this whole process of having breast cancer has affected us and some of the people in our lives. She began to tell me about how her sister acts as if she

does not have cancer. She said every time she speaks to her sister about her radiation treatments or her doctor's appointments her sister tends to brush it off as if nothing is wrong. She says she gets frustrated because she wants her sister to know that this really happening but she seems to ignore the whole thing. She continued to tell me that she just recently found out form her co-workers that when they ask her sister about her, her sister gets really upset and tells them that everything is okay and she gets really defensive with them. As I listened to her I could truly identify with what she was talking about. Not with my sister of course, she has been great through this whole process but with other people I have encountered. There have been people that have been extremely supportive then there were people that said, "Okay God can just take that away." I have spoken about this in a previous entry and I still feel the same way. I know God can just take it away and don't think I didn't want Him to, but if there is a message, a higher level or a place of insight that God is trying to bring me to then just taking this disease away would not have done it. God knows me and He knows what it will take to get me to a place in Him where I can help someone else. How can I be of help to someone if God has taken my burden away instantaneously, yet someone else has to persevere. I wouldn't know how to tell them to hang in there if I didn't have to. To me, that would be empty encouragement. Yes, this journey has been a whirlwind for me with its ups and downs but to know that I can give someone a true stable testimony of how God bought me through is a gift that keeps on giving.

Friday, November 9, 2012
Today I am very excited. I have only two more chemo treatments left then I can say good-riddance to this phase of my treatments. It has truly been a journey for me but I give God all the glory for everything. How great though Art!! I will also be returning to work in a couple of weeks and I am excited about that as well. I am slowly but surely getting back to some normalcy and it feels good…really good. Thank you Father for bringing me through.

Monday, November 12, 2012
Today I am really counting down till the day I can say farewell to my radiation treatments. Two more days and I will be out of there. I should be returning to work next week and I am anticipating on how many days I will take as half days. Until I work my way back into the full day workforce. I

have been ill this past weekend with my body feeling achy and my throat was extremely sore but I got through it thank God. I have to be careful of my surroundings and how I dress for the weather because the phlebotomist at the radiation clinic informed me that my white blood cells were still very low. The last thing I need is to get sick and not have anything to fight the illness with. So when I woke up with a sore throat it was quite concerning to me. However, today I am feeling well and in good spirits. Praise God!

Wednesday, November 14, 2012
Praise the Lord!! Today is the best day of my radiation. I cannot stress how elated I am. I woke up today looking forward to my treatment because I knew I would be walking out for the final time. Some of the women in the waiting area were all comparing their final dates as well and myself along with one other woman celebrated our final day today. After my treatment the nurses congratulated me and sent me off with well wishes and I in turn thanked them and let them know that was a pleasure meeting them and I hope I didn't have to see them again. At least not under these circumstances I added. As I walked into the dressing room to take off my gown I realized this chapter of my recovery went the

quickest, which I am happy about. I grabbed my clothes from the locker and began to charge all the while thinking about how great it was gonna be to have my life back. As I began to leave, I grabbed the gown I had just taken off and was about to put it back in the cubby that was assigned to my treatments. Cubby #1 was where I put my gown after every treatment and so out of habit I was about to put it back in its rightful place although I knew I wouldn't need it anymore, however, I quickly remembered that there wasn't a rightful place for my gown anymore so I gladly threw it into the bin with all the other gowns. I walked out the door of the North main radiology center feeling victorious and ready for my next phase. As I walked to my car, I didn't look back because there was nothing for me back there. It was finished!! As I pulled out of the parking lot, I felt as if I was leaving something behind that would not be missed but has served its purpose in my recovery. As I drove down North Main Street on my way home, I could only thank God for his grace and mercy because it is only through Him that I have been persevere.

Reflections

It seems so long ago that I made my first entry once I was diagnosed. I could not have imagined how far I would come through all of this. I could not have imagined how much God would allow me to take yet give me strength to overcome. I remember when I first heard the word cancer after my mammogram and sonogram, I wanted to just fall apart but little did I know that God is the glue that would hold me in place because there would be more in store for me than just a word. I remember all the appointments I had, all the picking and prodding, samples being taken and the blood work. My goodness the blood work!! I can't forget the bone scans, had several of those and about two eco-cardiograms as well. Then came the chemo and with that the complications began such as the blood in my lungs coagulating. What a nightmare!! Then my white blood cells diminishing, along with my red blood cells needing to be replenished, surgery more chemo, hair falling out, radiation, whew! This past year has truly been a whirlwind for me and I can only pray that I do not take this experience in vain but that God will use me to help someone else. As I continue to reflect on this experience, I can honestly say that in the midst of some of the worst times in my recovery,

God always sent someone to make me laugh or to encourage me. I can still picture the nurse in the operating room, singing and thinking she was good enough to try out for the X Factor, my oncology nurse Sandra, who has the smiling eyes and was always willing to share in my jokes or to share a funny story in my jokes or to share a funny story or two of her own, even some of the other patients would share their funny stories with me during our treatments but it was always when I was at a low point that God would use the people around me to lift my spirits. Oh yeah, I certainly can't forget my awesome church family. They have been such a blessing thru this whole process. I cannot begin to thank God enough for them and their prayers. My family has been really great as well. I really appreciate them coming out for my surgery and being as supportive as they have been. My sister Valerie has been phenomenal as my caregiver. I could not have asked for anyone better and I truly thank God for her and her servant's heart. My kids have been awesome and I thank God for their support and help through my recovery. To God be all the glory!!

Reflections Learned
I can remember asking God for me to be more like Him. That I want to have

compassion for others the way he has compassion. I remember the more I began to go deeper into my treatments, the more I began to have a heart for the people who were going through an illness. You never know what someone is going through until you walk in their shoes or even their path. I recall feeling sorry for myself and just having a pity party about my situation which was not the norm but for some reason it happened to rear its ugly head. As I was getting my chemo-treatment I struck up a conversation with a young woman who began to tell me about her fight with breast cancer. She finally let me know that she had to have a mastectomy because the cancer had consumed her whole breast. I remember feeling better after talking with her because my prognosis was a whole lot better and I was able to keep my breast. I know that God would not have me go through this for nothing, I know there is a higher realm that is awaiting me and I can only pray that I have passed the test in order to receive the blessing God has waiting for me. There is so much to tell about my journey, so much to share, yet I do not have words, I do not know how to express myself and quite frankly I think there are parts of my journey that I am not to disclose. There are situations God would have me keep to myself. Not for secrecy, but for my own personal growth and fulfillment. If it is the one thing I have learned it is to share with others what should be shared and to keep what is yours. This experience I have endured was given as a learning tool and has bought me closer to God. It has taught me that God is in the good and the bad, the highs and the lows, and He is in our sickness and health. I recall asking God why He would allow Satan to attach my body and God answered, "I told him he could attack your body but I never told him he would succeed in the end." I began to rejoice because today I am walking in victory and my health has improved beyond measure. Satan may have used his attacks for me but God turned it around for good. Satan may be a hard worker, but the Spirit of God works harder, longer, stronger and He does overtime. I can say today that I am a conqueror and more than an over comer and no matter what the circumstances of my existence; God always has a master plan. In the words of Bishop Jakes, I am to use a disaster and an adversity to develop my strength. In the end, I will realize how strong and resilient I really am. I want a stronger, better and more fulfilling life. To line the most highest and truest expression of myself as a human being. As I began to think more on my situation and looking forward to the end of my treatments, I learned from Bishop Jakes that I am not to stop where I am as though my final treatments were my destination, when in fact it could be transportation that brings me into that thing I was created to do. My situation is just a launching pad into the next dimension of my life. I discovered the pains and the burdens are not distractions. The greater the discretion the stronger the progression what is working against me is in fact working for me and the loss of my health was the discovery of my strength. Regardless of what comes my way, I do not want to disappoint God. I do not want to play the victim in all this but I want to be a good student, a good follower of the greatest teacher of all time. To achieve this, I must not become so busy with life as I use to be, thinking that because I was busy I was effective when in fact I was too busy for God and not hearing from Him the way I use to. Now with better insight from the Holy Spirit, and amore even-paced environment, I can listen for the instruction instead of returning to my hectic lifestyle and begging for direction. To God be the glory in all of this. He has truly been my rock and foundation, my fortress and my shield. He has been my bridge, my strength and my healing.

Yes, God is my healer. He is my "balm in Gilead."

After Thoughts

I returned to work on November 19, 2012. It was great to be back to work and feeling productive. I sat at my desk and was greeted with a balloon and flowers. My co-workers are the best. They have been so supportive and it makes my recovery all the more bearable. Our new location is pretty far, midway, Ma but the drive is pretty nice. I pop in a CD or hook up my smart phone turn on Pandora and just let in play. My supervisor is trying to get me closer to home so she is working with workplace accommodation to try and find me a position. Well, I look forward to what's in store at my new job location and I know God will work all things out for the good.

Monday, March 18, 2013
Today I found out I would be moving back to Rhode Island to work. Just me though. A position was found for me as a clerk working for second level managers. Only thing is there is no overtime. Ugh! I like my overtime but my health is more important. And if I should get sick I will be able to collect TDI. I will be starting April 1 and I am excited. Training will be

in providence but my office will be in Warwick.

Monday, April 1, 2013
Training is going good and there is a lot to learn. My office gave me a farewell party the Friday before and my Supervisor Karen cried when I was leaving. She has been outstanding through this whole thing and I thank God she was the one that started with me though all this. I have about a week or two left of training then it will be time to go out on my own. I now there is a lot to learn but I would prefer to learn by doing rather than sitting behind someone and looking over their shoulder. Lord, please hold me up through this.

Monday, April 15, 2013
Today I start vacation and I am so looking forward to it. I have developed this cough for a few weeks now and it is pretty annoying. I have the chills also so it could be the flu. Nonetheless, I will be going to the doctor's office tomorrow to have it checked out. Gee-whiz, this is my vacation, can't I get some rest?

Wednesday, April 17, 2013
Okay so here I sit for the second time at the clinic. Yesterday, after an exam and x-rays the doctor said he

wanted to come back to the clinic because of my results. I was concerned because he called me at 6:30 p.m. he said he found nodules on my lungs so he was concerned because of my cancer history. He asked me if I wanted him to call my doctor and I said yes, since he can explain the situation better than I can. I was given a prescription yesterday, an inhaler to help with the shortness of breathing. What in the world is in store for me? God only knows.

Wednesday, April 17, 2013
My doctor calls me and asks me a few questions about my symptoms. I let him know about my shortness of breath and the cough I had been having for about a month. He says he wants me to go for a CT scan the next day and for me to see him on that Friday. The appointments are made and all the while I am thinking that maybe the doctor at the walk-in clinic is wrong. There probably is nothing wrong but he just wants to take precaution just in case. Then something downed on me. My oncology doctor called me himself. He "never" does that. Usually he would have the nurse practitioner or one of the secretaries that handles the appointments do that. Oh boy!! I'm trying not to think the worse. I know my God is bigger than anything I may

have to endure, and yes, I need Big God right now.

Friday, April 19, 2013
I went to the doctor today and for some reason I wasn't too concerned as I thought. Maybe because I had psyched myself in the hopes that the doctor at the walk-in clinic was wrong. As I begin to undress for my exam I wondered if Dr. S would be long at all. Well, he wasn't. He quickly examines me and tells me he doesn't hear anything in my lungs. That relieves me because the doctor at the walk in clinic said he did. Dr. S tells me to get dress so we can talk so I quickly put my clothes on. When he returns to the room I quickly inform him that I see he has that "face" of concern. He says yeah he does and he proceeds to tell me in his most concerned yet gentle manner that his worst fears have been confirmed. The cancer has re-occurred and it was in my lungs. I was saddened but not as much as I thought because I automatically began to think about how I beat it the last time. So I asked him was it curable and he shook his head and said, "No!"

Sunday, April 21, 2013
Had to take a breather from that last entry. Was quite a shock to the system. I was very taken aback by his

response and I believe it showed by me taking a deep breath and the wide-eyed look on my face. He informed of a combination of chemo drugs that can be administered along with what I am already being given. There is a good change these spots on my lungs can be shrunk to a level of being put under control. The success rate is more than half. So the doctor felt confident of my chances of being successful with this drug. We agree I will begin my new treatments on the scheduled Friday of my ordinary appointment. So what was a 45 minute treatment would now become a 3 ½ to 4 hour treatment. He begins to explain to me the types of medications that will be administered and wrote them down for me to research them and if I have any questions to call him. I appreciate my doctor for doing that and for giving me the opportunity to make sure I feel comfortable and confident with what he is doing to treat my disease. As I leave, my doctor hugs me and says that he is sorry for not having any better news but I thank him for his concern and his help and insight that I feel he has always been willing to share with me without my always having to guess or pry from him during this whole journey. After making my new appointments, I share my findings with my sister Val who becomes nervous and asks if it will, in her own words, "take me out of here." I shake my head no and dismiss her question as just her being in shock and not having anything else to say. Sometimes you just have to encourage yourself. When I get home I begin to call my other sisters and my aunt because they know about the x-rays and my appointment so they wanted to know the results. They were very supportive as always and my sister Deneen cried as if she was already at my funeral. It was expected so I wasn't surprised at all. I informed my oldest son James and he was concerned by saying he wasn't worried about it being incurable because he knows I'm not going anywhere. He said it with such surety that if it wasn't for my own faith I could have drawn off his confidence alone. I didn't tell my son Tevin but will wait till' later. I need him to concentrate on his studies at school. He is about to graduate and is just getting his grades up to par. What a journey and rollercoaster ride this has been for me. God has been there all the time to sustain me even through my tears and frustrations. He is so awesome and I know He is not through with me yet.

Friday, April 26, 2013
Today I had my first full chemo treatment. I had a visit with my

doctor first and asked him some questions about my condition. I looked up the conditions as lung cancer but my doctor told me that my breast cancer had traveled to my lungs so the questions I had were null and void. My cancer is Her2 cancer and is pretty aggressive and can travel throughout the body. He also informed me they found a spot on my bone near my spine so I have to go for a bone scan and will probably have to go for brain scan as well because it can travel there also. After my visit, more appointments are made and I make my way to the third floor for chemo. My nurse Sandra is there and she and I always have a laugh. Last time she and I saw each other we were talking about cleaning our fruits and vegetables. She said she didn't clean her fruit when she ate it and I was pretty taken aback. I told her there were germs and bacteria on the fruits and veggies but she just said she didn't think about it. SO when she saw me today she informed me that she went to buy some apples the other day and saw the guy in the produce section running his hands over the apples as he is filling the bin and she automatically thought about me. She said she bought the apples and when she got home she washed them with soap and water like I told her I did. We laughed about the whole thing and that just set the tone for the day ahead. I told Sandra that I was praying for her when she told me about not washing her food. So now she knows. As I sat in my chair to begin my treatments there was a woman beside me and as soon as I sat down I said hello and she said she heard me say that I was praying for someone. I automatically knew I was in the company of a fellow believer in Christ and all was well with my soul. I never got her name but we had a great conversation about church and our faith and it was great to share ourselves and experiences. My nurse Sandra comes in with my pre-meds that I get before my chemo and we share more laughs. She looks at me with curiosity and asks if I ever have a time where I am sad or down because whenever I am around I am always upbeat and jovial. I let her know I have my moments but they are very few and a lot of times I am usually happy regardless of the situation. She seems content with my response and begins to hook me up to my first medication, Benadryl. Taking my pill is one thing, having it go straight to your system is another. I remember eating a sandwich my sister Val packed for me and drinking a juice. I remember Val sitting next to me, my words slurring as I was talking and asking the nurse is that the Benadryl taking effect and she said yes as she began to laugh at me. I close my eyes and wake up 2 ½ hours later.

Sunday, April 28, 2013
Two days now after chem. And I have yet to be sick with nausea. I have been taking my medication as prescribed and it has been a blessing to be able to get up and feel good in the morning and throughout the day. Today I will have the elders of the church pray over me for my healing. I know God is more than willing so I am moving on His word in the book of James 5:14-15 where it states, "Is anyone of you sick? He should call the elders of the church to pray for him and anoint him with oil in the name of the Lord. And the prayer offered in faith will make the sick person well; the Lord will raise him up. If he has sinned he will be forgiven." Praise God!!

Saturday, May 11, 2013
SO much has happened since my last entry. I found out that my oldest sister Princess has pancreatic cancer and has had it for a while. Lord I know you can heal her like you did my breast cancer and I pray you will give her strength beyond measure. Give her a testimony for others to be encouraged by. I went for a bone scan yesterday and would you believe I fell asleep on

the table during the test? Unbelievable!! I believe the tests will come back negative and that God will handle all things. Right now there is so much on my mind that I cannot tell it all. One thing I do know is that motherhood seems to be more challenging than my condition right now. As a mom I have a passion to see my children succeed in life and when I see the enemy trying to sway them away from the things of God I go into "fight" mode. God has answered my prayer and has allowed Tevin to be able to go to a charter school rather than the school across the street so I am so psyched about that. These teenage years are not the best years but I have to make it through and give it my best as God has given me a job to do. Lord help me to go further in what it is you would have me to do with my children. In Jesus name; Amen!!

Monday, May 20, 2013
I had my second chemo treatment and for some reason I am feeling sluggish. I will preserve today and try to get through it. There is so much on my mind right now financially, physically and emotionally but I give it all to God and ask for His unending wisdom and guidance. There just seems to be a heaviness on me right now and yes, I want it removed. I know God would not

have me feel this way so I do not want to dwell on whatever it is but I want it gone. For now I will start my day anew, as God's mercies are new every day and I thank Him for that. How refreshing...

Monday, June 17, 2013
It's been a while since my last entry but because I live such a predictable life, at least from my stand-point, there really wasn't much to tell until now. Last week my sister Val and I went to Atlanta to be with our other siblings. Our visit was also at the request of our oldest sister Princess (Adorn) who is suffering from chronic pancreatic cancer. I almost didn't make the trip because I had to run home to get my luggage that I had forgotten then upon arrival to the airport. I realized I forgot my photo I.D. through it all; I was able to make the trip. We stayed at a spa-resort where my sister Deneen works and boy was this place fabulous. The stay was overnight but the time spent was priceless. The following day we all took pictures and for some reason I decided to take the pictures without my head-concerning. "YUCK." I want my hair back, but I want my health first. The pics came out good nonetheless, and then we all went to stay at Deneen's house. Saturday was a blessed event. My

sister Princess was finally baptized. Praise God! This was something she has always wanted to do even though situations would occur and block her form doing it. I guess the reality of her condition finally compelled her, or maybe even scared her into making it happen. I thank God for His grace and mercy once again and sparing her life long enough to be able to give her life to Him and to be baptized. Saturday before our departure we went to an awesome cookout at our cousin Anissa's house. It's always good to see family and it was good to see everyone enjoying themselves, cracking jokes and talking about old times. Oh yeah, I must say a quick prayer, "Lord please help my Aunt Delores realize that you have delivered her from drinking so she does not need to carry that Royal Crown bag around her wrist with her personal belongings in it. Help her find a nice pocket book or handbag so she can move forward to the next phase in her deliverance, in Jesus name, Amen." I had to say this prayer because we were trying to convince my aunt that carrying around this bag was not a good idea. Not to mention we were told by her daughter-in-law she takes it to church, yes, church and sings and claps her hands all the while the bag is swinging back and forth. Unbelievable! Gotta love her though! Sunday, while in the Atlanta airport on our way home, I became winded and couldn't walk the length of the airport because they moved our flight. I had to be put in a wheelchair and taken to the gate. The young lady who worked for Delta that pushed me in the chair was very nice and she was also a praying woman who said a quick prayer for me after helping me board the plane. Through my whole trip in Atlanta I had a cough and a shortness of breath and I believe it was due to the humidity. When I returned home my doctor said I could use my inhaler if that should happen again. My trip was great but I miss traveling with my kids. We always have a good time. I know God will provide the trip for me and my kids and I can speak for them when I say it will be Universal Orlando. Can't wait to get on those rides.

Sunday, July 21, 2013
Friday I had two appointments at the Breast Health Center. The first was with Dr. S. I have to admit I have really grown to trust and value his opinion regarding my condition and his presence and bedside manner is rather comforting as well. I had taken a CAT Scan on July 16 so my appointment was to get the results. Dr. S informed me the scan showed the spots on my lungs were shrinking; however he wished they

would have disappeared. He let me know that although they hadn't disappeared, it showed progress so he wanted to take me off the chemo drug and continue my treatment with the lesser drugs Herceptin and Pertuzumab. He said these two drugs would still be 30% effective in my treatment. I was glad to hear that I wasn't getting the chemo anymore and that my system can go back to being as normal as possible. My hair will grow back, I will not have to take my steroid meds and I will not have to take a **Lunastar**?? Shot after chemo. Yes, Friday was a good day. Afterwards I had chemo, oh my new chemo treatment at 11:30 a.m. and all went well as usual. However, I must admit as happy as I was to not have the chemo meds, I did miss not getting the Benadryl. Boy that was some good stuff. Oh well, can't have everything. Thank you God for answering my prayers. My healing is not far away…

Saturday, August 3, 2013
The summer is flying by and I am trying to hold out as much of it as possible. I'm not ready for the snow, the cold or anything else that is associated with the winter. However, I am ready for a change in my job and I know God has heard me. Thursday, I found out that there are 48 positions open with the company and boy am I happy. It will be

closer to my home and Tevin's school will not be too far either. Not to mention there will be a significant pay-raise along with the position. There will be challenges as far as studying for the test and I have to pass a seven week class as well but I am relying on God for the whole thing. My spirit is ready for this and I want God to lead me and guide me the whole way. I look forward to what He has for me because He has never let me down. Although I disappoint Him daily. Thank you Father for your everlasting love, kindness and mercy.

Saturday, August 31, 2013
It's been a while since my last entry. I have come to realize that the longer I fight this battle with cancer, the less my entries are. I believe it's because I am into a routine now and there truly isn't much to say. Of course, I can write about God's grace and mercy on a daily basis, but sometimes I just let Him know that personally. I pray whoever reads this knows that God is already the center of my life and the reason I live. God guides me daily and though sometimes I go my own way, He always redirects me. My last entry stated that I wanted to apply for another position on my job and I did. However, I didn't pass the test. I was a little bummed out at

first because I really wanted that job but I know God always has a "ram in the bush." I will trust and believe that He has a more excellent plan for me than what I wanted. Also, yesterday I had a doctor's appointment. It is always good to see Dr. S. I always mention how wonderful his bedside manner is and I stand by that even now. I found out that there was no end to my chemo treatments so I guess I have this to look forward to for a while. But I must remember that the diagnosis is what man says. What does God say? He says that, "Healing is the children's bread." He also said, "For I am the Lord that heals you." (Exodus 15:26) He is also the God who forgives sins and heals diseases (Psalm 103:3) there is so much more and I know my total and complete healing is just a little more faith away. Thank you Father. I intend to keep pushing toward that total faith that brings total healing, total deliverance and total surrender. Praise God!

Sunday, October 6, 2013
It's been a whole month since my last entry and I have begun to realize that I am getting sick and tired of being sick and tired. This all began as something I wanted to share with others but now it is something I am ready to be done with. The cancer is continuing

to spread in my lungs so now I am on two types of inhalers and cough medicines that suppress the constant cough I have. I am about to be out of work for a while, I'll need a handicapped decal because I can't walk far. I have begun a new type of chemo that I pray will work in my favor and I have realized that I am slowly becoming short tempered and bitter. I am trying not to go there because my recovery is hanging in the balance so staying close to God and the positive people He has put in my life is crucial. It is so easy to become complacent and just roll with the circumstances but that is not what I want. I do not want to be complacent but I do want to be active in my recovery. This is not how I want my story to end! I am and have so much more than what I have been dealt. Sometimes I feel it's so unfair for this to have happened to me but I know that is a state of mind I cannot entertain for long because for whatever reason, God has a job, a mission for me to complete and I want to be at my post no matter what! Regardless of the chemo, regardless of the coughing, regardless of the vomiting, regardless of the doctors' visits, regardless of the doctors warning to have my affairs in order, regardless of all the medications, I intend to be at my post no matter what!! -Amen-

Monday, November 11, 2013
Today as I was reading my devotional I was enlightened and encouraged. I read James 5 and it was about persevering. This encouraged me because I know regardless of how I feel I must continue to go on in Christ Jesus. I must be mindful of what God would have me to do during this time in my life. I must be mindful of the type of influence I have regarding others which is very important because regardless of my illness I still carry the Spirit of Christ within me so I must properly represent Him at all times. To God be the glory…Amen.

Thursday, November 28, 2013
Happy Thanksgiving! I have so much to be thankful for. Mainly the family and friends that God has put into my life and the love of God that keeps me strong and going forward from day to day. Yesterday I had a doctor's appointment with Dr. S and he informed me that the spots on my lungs are not spreading any further and have stabilized. He let me know on another form of chemo because he wants to see the spots shrinking. I won't be having chemo this Friday but will be awaiting the results of my blood work so I can find out which route I will be going with this new chemo. He even told me I may be going to Boston for treatment if

necessary. Whatever it takes and whatever God has in store for me I will gladly follow. I know there are good things at the end of this journey and I want it all. Thank you Father for the strength to endure it all. I pray I am making you proud and bringing glory to your name. That's all that matters!!

Tuesday, December 17, 2013
I had my first round of chemo Dec. 6, 2013 and it went well. I was tired afterwards but went to my church Christmas party and stayed longer than I anticipated. However, I paid for it later. I was in bed until Monday morning. I guess I overtaxed my body, so I know not to do that anymore. Today as I was reading my daily devotion I came across a passage about over- working yourself to the point that you neglect your body. That hit home because before I was diagnosed that is exactly what I was doing. Work, work, work, that was all I did. My devotional warned that because of this. It will cause the break-down of the body which should be the temple of the Holy Spirit and for that we will have to answer to God for. Will I have to answer to God for neglecting my body? Will I have to give an account for working so much and not giving more time to Him and myself? Is my condition a result of my past actions

or is it a test that God only gives to His strongest people? Father please forgive me for my past actions that may have caused the breakdown of my body and strengthen me now and forever more. Amen...

Remembrance of Kathryn's preparation for going Home by her sister Valerie

Wednesday, December 25, 2013
"Merry Christmas!" Happy Birthday, My Lord. Thank you for allowing us another holiday with my sisters Kathy and Princess. At 7:30 AM I call my sisters to wish them a Merry Christmas. At 8:30 AM I pick up the phone to call Kathy; the phone rang in my hand. Kathy said, "Val I hurt so badly. Meet me at the hospital." As I ran to my bedroom to get ready, I remember praying "Father the devil is a liar! Not on your most Holy Day will he prevail, over your daughter (Matthew 8:26)". When I got to the hospital, Kathy was hospitalized. It seems that two of the tumors in her lungs had begun to grown along with her having pneumonia, bronchitis and asthma. I asked myself, "Father God, how much more can my sister take? I'm so scared. Help me Heavenly father Kathy's faith never weaver but mines is all over the place."

As I looked into my sister's beautiful brown eyes I saw faith and love for our Heavenly father. I saw in her lovely eyes, not yet Val not today. As the days went by, I couldn't help but reflect on Kathy's faith how dedicated, thankful and grateful she was. She

seems to always be at constant peace.
I wonder if her illness ever bothered
her, if she even cried, got angry, if
she had temper tantrum, what did she
think, how she felt, was she scared. I
remember asking her if she had any
doubts, Kathy replied, "Val all I have
is my faith. It's all in God's hands
and His will be done."

Sunday, December 29, 2013
Today is my nephew Eric's birthday.
Kathy and I talk about our mother;
today would have been her birthday
also. We laughed and traded childhood
stories about mom. I told Kathy a
funny story about mom and I, she
laughed so hard that she had to have a
respiratory treatment. It felt good to
see her laugh like that, uncontrollably
laughter as I think about it; it was
pretty funny then and now. I say,
"Sorry for causing you to have a
respiratory treatment."

Monday, December 30, 2013
Today I felt pretty comfortable leaving
Kat, as I affectionately called her,
overnight at the hospital. Normally I
stay with her until she is discharged.
This morning I woke with a sad heart as
I was leaving to go back to the
hospital. An overwhelming sadness
overtook me as I began praying for my
sister. A lot of tears ran down my

face. I prayed for her healing to come home, for her children, I don't know, I just prayed. In the midst of my praying, God revealed to me Kathy standing in front of the local Hospital. I felt at peace and I knew she was coming home.

<u>Wednesday, January 1, 2014</u>
What a blessed New Year it is Kathy is home!!! Thank you Father. Thank you for seeing us through this past year. The Medical Center decided to give Kathy her chemo treatment before her discharge. I was happy about that because I didn't want to bring her back out in this cold weather, once I got her home. Beside we were getting a snow storm tonight. I was worried about her respiratory equipment that had to be delivered to the house before she got there.
Kathy's message that day was, "Happy New Year to all my family and friends. May the New Year be the year of complete overflow for you and your families as I make the same request for me and my family. Stay focused, be blessed and may God continue to shine His love and peace upon you."
I packed up all of Kat's belongings and helped get her dressed.

I did a mental check:
   ✓ Medication: call to pharmacy

- ✓ Everything packed
- ✓ Dress very warmly – now it's starting to snow
- ✓ Chemo treatment done
- ✓ Respiratory treatment – done visiting nurses 2x per week
- ✓ Respiratory equipment – delivered phlebotomy coming next week
- ✓ Wheelchair

And away we go! Wait "STOP"! Kathy needs a shot before her discharge and her insurance won't pay for it while she is a patient at the hospital. The insurance will only pay for the shot as we outpatient, and the hospital can't give her the shot as an outpatient. I said to myself, "Are you freaking kidding me"! As you know though God is truly an awesome God because Kathy got her shot! As we arrive home, the respiratory equipment tech is waiting outside. The equipment tech set up the machines and connected Kat to the first one which is 4 in-all. He walked Kat and me through everything. The central respiratory machine was placed in the dining room with a fifty foot cord so Kat could move around the house easily. She had to have oxygen 2 ½ Lit 24/7. A 200lb tank was placed in her bedroom in case we lost power during the snow storm.

Saturday, January 4, 2014
As I was staying with Kathy at her house, we lost heat and two days later we had eleven inches of snow and it was only fifteen degree. I called Kathy's oldest son James to go by my house and pick up three electric heaters. When James returned, we wrapped Kathy up in many blankets and put the biggest heater next to her. Though I wanted to take her to my house, I was not comfortable unplugging her machines or taking her out in that bad weather. The heat came back on two hours later and everything turned out fine. We know God is in control.

As the days of January rolled by, Kathy and I settled into a daily routine. Our routine consisted of me working nights and spending my days with her. Kathy would always say, "Val go lay in my bed and get some sleep. I know you're tired." I just couldn't sleep surpass my beautiful sister needing me.

Kathy loved when her granddaughter Amiah would come over. Kathy loves that little girl and Kathy was her Diva. Amiah turned five on New Year's Day could not understand why Diva didn't come to her birthday party.

Kathy tried to explain to her that she was sick that is why she couldn't make it. "Why didn't you tell me I would have brought you some cake and came over to help you", Amiah said. That night Amiah wanted to stay the night with her Diva, but couldn't. Her father James tried to explain to her that she can't because Diva was sick. But all Amiah knew was that her Diva was sick and that's why she had to stay the night so she can help her get better.

Friday, January 24, 2014
Today started out cloudy, gray and very cold. I fixed breakfast for Amiah and Kathy, though Kathy didn't eat much this morning. James was rushing out the house to take Tevin and Amiah to school this morning. He kissed his mother goodbye, Amiah kissed her Diva goodbye, and Tevin ran straight to the door. Kathy called him back for her kiss. She said "boy come give me my kiss, it might be the last one."

After everyone left, I went to wash up the morning dishes. I then checked the weather, I was hoping James would be back soon to clean the snow off Kathy's car. I remember asking Kat what time it was, she turned and said "10:17 a.m." I decided to sit for a few minutes because her appointment wasn't until 12:30 p.m. Kathy said that she really didn't feel like going to chemo today that she was extremely tired. I told her she had to go and dosed off to sleep. Kathy said, "Val, can you get my blue pants so we can go. I got her pants and as she was putting them on she became tired and short of breath. She asked me to help her put her paints on which I did. She became extremely short of breath and wanted to sit down so she can catch her breath. I increased her oxygen from 2L to 3L. I asked her if she was okay and she started laughing and said now she had to go pee, we both began laughing. I got her computer chair and rolled her in the bathroom and that's when she told me she wasn't breathing. I asked if she was short of breath and she said, "NO I CAN'T BREATH." She started crying and I ran and dialed 911, unlocked and opened her front door, and ran back to the bathroom to try to help her by increasing oxygen to 4L. The ambulance came and rushed Kathy out. I called her oldest son James and he picked me up and we rushed to the hospital. In a matter of an hour Kathy was placed on life support. The doctors tried talking to me about turning off the machine. I know that this is not what Kathy would have wanted because we talked about it a lot and she said if this was to ever happen she wanted to be resuscitated. The Doctors did just that and placed her back on life support. My son picked up Kathy's youngest son Tevin from school. They finally let James, Tevin and I in to the room to see Kathy. They told us that she wouldn't be able to respond or hear us but that prove to be wrong. As I was holding her hand I called her name and told her I was here and she turned her head and looked at me for a few seconds. I told James to talk to her and as he talked to her, she turned her head towards him and the tears rolled down the side of her face. Tevin said, "Mommy I'm here", at that point Kathy started fighting and bucking the machine, she tried to open her eyes, her tears rolled down the side of her face much more and even faster.

The hospital moved Kathy to the MICU to run more tests to find out what caused her to stop breathing and her heart to start slowing down. Though a filter was placed in her a year ago, her body was creating so many blood clots that the filter could not stop them all. Some of the blood clots went to her heart and lungs which caused her to stop breathing. I remember sitting there holding Kathy's hand kissing her face and singing The Storm is Over. As I was singing both her Pastors was praying.

6:45 PM my beautiful God fearing sister, Kathryn Brown's journey here on Earth was complete.

Many may say Conquerer? Well Kathy has conquered her journey here on Earth and I am sure she will conquer whatever journey that God has in store for her in the future.

Amen!

In Remembrance of our sister, our mother, Kathryn Brown

Kathy,

My sister, my friend… God's Child
Fierce, loyal, loving … God's Child
Disciplined, faithful, obedient… God's Child
Strong, intelligent, generous… God's Child
I miss you, I love you, truly you are deserving of hearing from Our Lord: "well done…good and faithful servant."
Love Jody

Kathy,

A woman who brought sunshine into any room she walked into. Kathy was fighter who fought to the end. Her qualities are worth imitating and her smile can light up anyone's life. I will miss you; until I see you again.
Love Roxanne

Kathy,

Every day that I'm here I pray. Every day the way I live, isn't God's will so I cry. But this Morning I seen you. It happened so fast I felt chills and my heart skipped a beat. So I said to

myself Kathy was that you if so I'm glad you're here. How much I miss you saying to us: No Sir!! Your laughter, Your smile, always having a praise for someone (ha-ha) how you would say you need to find Jesus. This Morning I want thank you little Sister for all laughter, joy, and the pain we all been through. Until we meet again, I'm Loving You and Missing you. The Lord has blessed you and he has YOU.
Love Adorn

Kathy,

My beloved baby sister as I'm sitting here trying to write a farewell and final message to you the tears are just running down my face my hands can't hold the pen and my heart is so heavy and painful. I find myself asking God how do you say anything final to someone you still have not allowed to come to an end how do you say farewell to someone that is so so still alive in your soul I still talk to you as if you were right here I still hear your laughter I still feel your touch then I get so sad I just want to scream. I can't believe no matter how hard I try that you are gone I have those last words you said to me Deneen, I'm having an awesome time with the Lord this morning early will I seek Him, when I read that text from you for a brief moment I smiled I thank God and a calm peacefulness came over me. Because I felt that you knew and that she was okay with the decision that God had laid upon you that should work here on earth was done. But even now I still cannot muster up anything farewell or final to say to you but what I can say is Lord I miss you so my love still grows for you each and every day and there is not one day that goes by since the day you received your wings that I don't talk to you or think about you so farewell or goodbyes I can't do but what I can say is see you later alligator and after while crocodile until we meet again I'll keep talking to you loving you laughing with you and always always cherishing our bond. PS I love you. **Love Deneen**

Kathy,

I had to ask myself: Am I selfish to say I wasn't ready? Am I selfish to say I needed more time with you? Am I selfish to say I need to hear your voice and your laughter? Am I selfish to say I need to see your smile? Am I selfish to say I just need at least one more vacation with you?
I asked God: Why was she taken so soon, she still had a lot to do here on

Earth? Why couldn't you leave her here with her family who needed her, who valued her opinion and admired her strength and whit? Why would you take her knowing I couldn't handle it, how heavy my heart is, knowing I still cry silently? Then a song came on and sang: "Heaven Couldn't Wait for You… so go home, go home." In that moment my questions and fears was answered. God needed you more and I know you are okay and in God's hands now. I love you, I miss you, and I can't wait to see you again!

Love Anissa

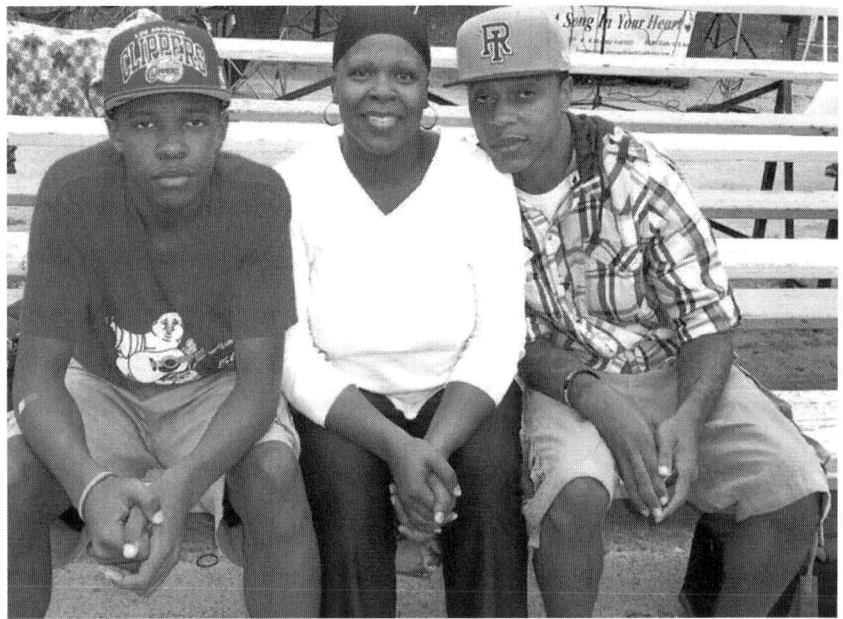

Kathy and her sons: Tevin (left) and James (right)

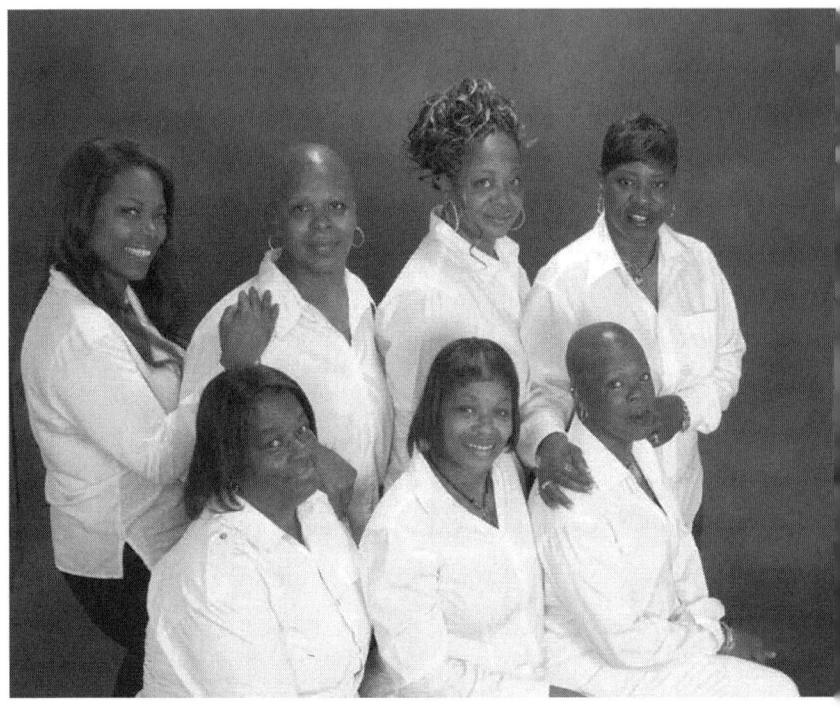

**Top left to right: Anissa, Kathy, Jody, and Deneen
Bottom left to right: Roxanne, Adorn (Princess), Valerie**

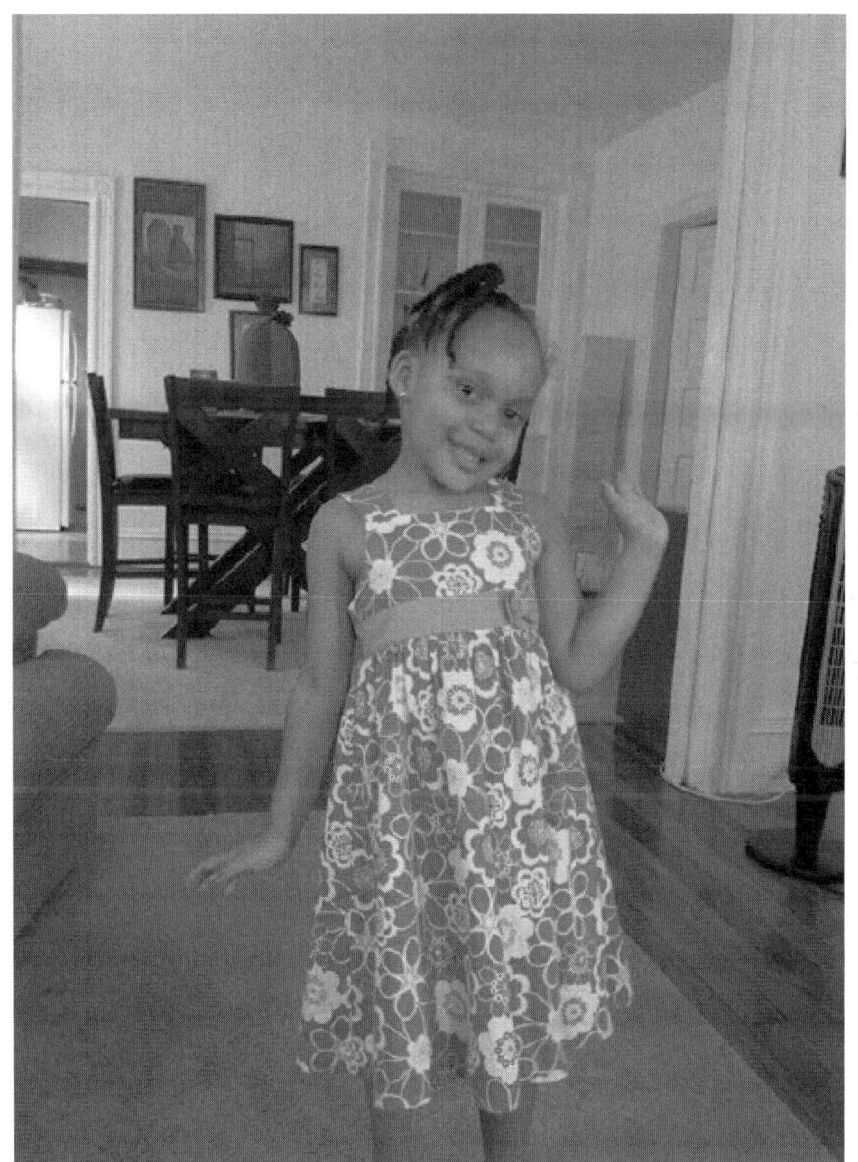
Kathy's granddaughter Amiah

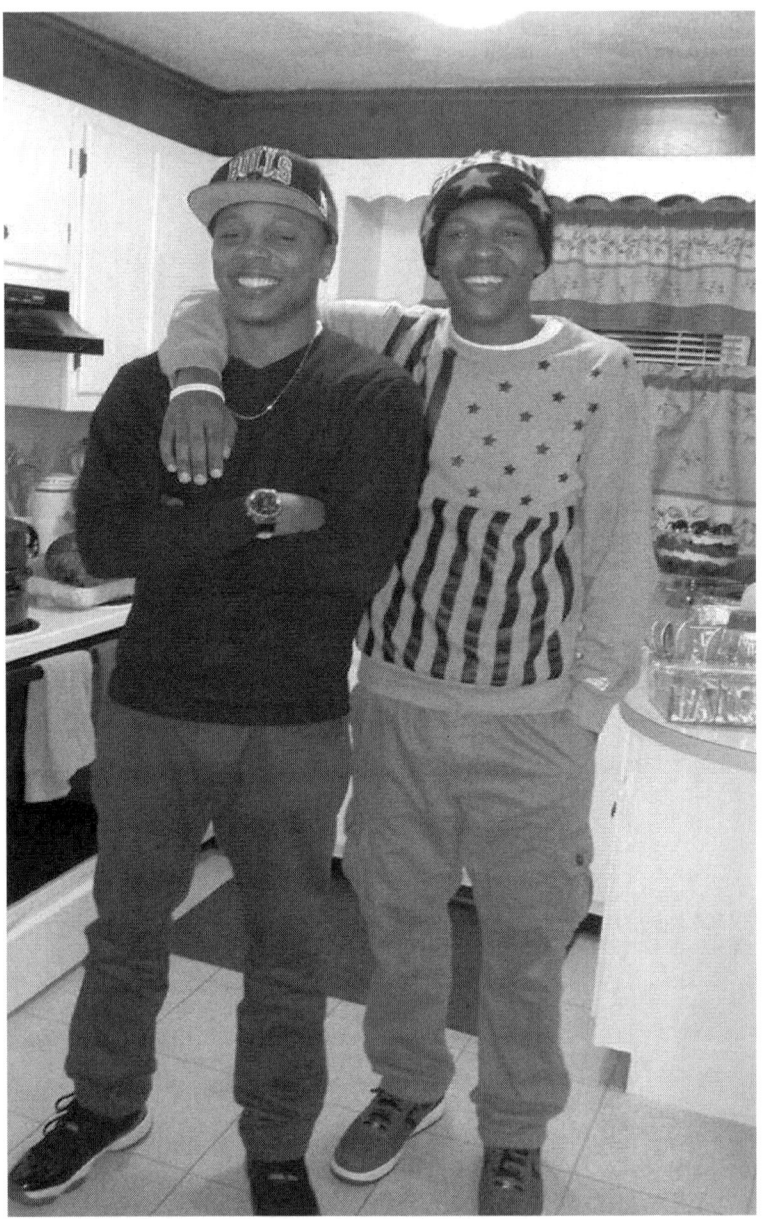

James and Tevin

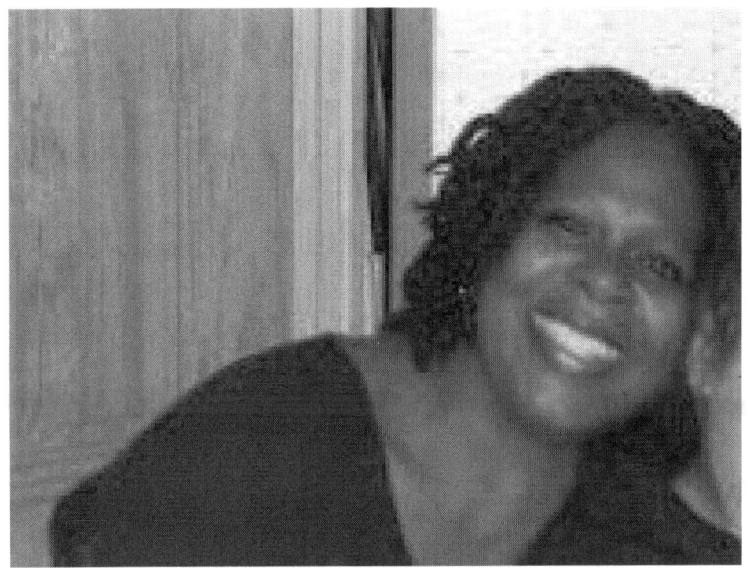

Beautiful Kathy